Translation Prac

Translation Practices Explained is a series of coursebooks designed to help self-learners and teachers of translation. Each volume focuses on a specific aspect of professional translation practice, in many cases corresponding to actual courses available in translator-training institutions. Special volumes are devoted to well consolidated professional areas, such as legal translation or European Union texts; to areas where labour-market demands are currently undergoing considerable growth, such as screen translation in its different forms; and to specific aspects of professional practices on which little teaching and learning material is available, the case of editing and revising, or electronic tools. The authors are practising translators or translator trainers in the fields concerned. Although specialists, they explain their professional insights in a manner accessible to the wider learning public.

These books start from the recognition that professional translation practices require something more than elaborate abstraction or fixed methodologies. They are located close to work on authentic texts, and encourage learners to proceed inductively, solving problems as they arise from examples and case studies.

Each volume includes activities and exercises designed to help self-learners consolidate their knowledge; teachers may also find these useful for direct application in class, or alternatively as the basis for the design and preparation of their own material. Updated reading lists and website addresses will also help individual learners gain further insight into the realities of professional practice.

Dorothy Kelly
Series Editor

Medical Translation Step by Step

Learning by Drafting

Vicent Montalt
Maria González Davies

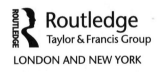

LONDON AND NEW YORK

First published 2007 by St. Jerome Publishing

Published 2014 by Routledge
2 Park Square, Milton Park, Abingdon, Oxon OX14 4RN
711 Third Avenue, New York, NY 10017, USA

Routledge is an imprint of the Taylor & Francis Group, an informa business

Notices
Knowledge and best practice in this field are constantly changing. As new research and experience broaden our understanding, changes in research methods, professional practices, or medical treatment may become necessary.

Practitioners and researchers must always rely on their own experience and knowledge in evaluating and using any information, methods, compounds, or experiments described herein. In using such information or methods they should be mindful of their own safety and the safety of others, including parties for whom they have a professional responsibility.

To the fullest extent of the law, neither the Publisher nor the authors, contributors, or editors, assume any liability for any injury and/or damage to persons or property as a matter of products liability, negligence or otherwise, or from any use or operation of any methods, products, instructions, or ideas contained in the material herein.

ISBN 13: 978-1-900650-83-0 (pbk)
ISSN 1470-966X (*Translation Practices Explained*)

Typeset by
Print-tech India

British Library Cataloguing in Publication Data
A catalogue record of this book is available from the British Library

Library of Congress Cataloging-in-Publication Data
   Montalt, Vicent.
   Medical translation step by step : learning by drafting / Vicent Montalt, Maria
      Gonzalez Davies.
      p. cm. -- (Translation practices explained)
      Includes bibliographical references and index.
      ISBN 1-900650-83-5 (pbk. : alk. paper)
      1. Medicine--Translating. I. Gonzalez Davies, Maria. II. Title.

   R118.6.M66 2007
   610--dc22
                                        2006101395

Contents

*Documentary research for these chapters was carried out by Balma Forés and Maite Sánchez, both of Universitat Jaume I, Castelló, Spain.

List of Figures

Chapter 5

Chapter 6

Chapter 7

Acknowledgments

At every stage in the production of this book the support I have received from Margaret Miller, a dear friend of many years, has been invaluable. She acted as a sounding board for my ideas and the many discussions we had, particularly in the early stages, helped me to clarify my vision of the whole work. Later she read and revised several drafts of chapters 1, 2, 3, 4, 6 and 7, and her perceptive comments and suggestions on content, presentation and style, and her wise counsel, have saved me from many errors. Any that still remain are, of course, my own. I acknowledge her contribution with gratitude.

I also appreciate the contribution of Morten Pilegaard, Jan Engberg, Peter Steffensen, Peter Kastberg, and Patrick Leroyer, of the Aarhus School of Business, and Rafael Aleixandre, of the Universitat de València, who read and commented on chapters 6 and 7.

I would also like to thank Balma Fores and Maite Sánchez, of the Universitat Jaume I, for their feedback on a number of chapters as well as their contribution to chapters 2 and 3 as research assistants in the last stage of the process.

Special thanks go to the students and teachers of the postgraduate course on medical translation <http://www.tradmed.uji.es> as well as to my colleagues at the GENTT research project <http://www.gentt.uji.es> – both at the Universitat Jaume I – from whom I have received useful feedback with regard to the practice and research of medical translation.

Last but not least I wish to thank my family –especially my mother Maria Amparo and my father Vicent–, Merxe and my friends for their unconditional support.

Vicent Montalt
Universitat Jaume I

I would like to thank Dr Josep Enric Boada whose inspiration, help and love for the world of medicine have been crucial in my career. A special mention goes to all those medical practitioners I have met along the years who understand the work of medical translators and are always willing to give up part of their time to help us improve our work.

I also have to thank Dr Eva Espasa and Dr Víctor Obiols from the University of Vic for excellent teaching ideas and support with medical translation subjects, as well as my students of so many years at the Department of Translation at the University of Vic.

Finally, I wish to mention that my contribution to the book has been financed with a grant awarded by the DURSI (*Departament d'Universitats per a la Recerca i Societat de la Informació*, Generalitat de Catalunya, DOGC nº 3812, 2003MQD) and the interuniversity research group GRACTLE .

Maria González Davies
Universitat de Vic and
Universitat Ramon Llull

We wish to acknowledge the helpful guidance of Dorothy Kelly as general editor of the *Translation Practices Explained* series.

How to use this book: underlying principles

This book deals with the basics of medical translation and with learning how to translate medical texts. It is, therefore, a book that presents facts and information on medical translation and guidelines on how to perform successfully. As part of the series *Translation Practices Explained*, the book explores the processes in medical translation to give a broad understanding of the topic and help to improve translation skills. We focus on three main aspects medical writing, translation practice and the exploration of learning paths to achieve a more effective product. There is little literature with this orientation and coursebooks to complement teaching material or to advance self-study are much needed in educational programmes worldwide.

Our preliminary questions have been: What is medical translation? Are there different kinds of medical translation? How can medical translation be learnt? Can we design helpful tasks to improve the necessary skills? To explore these points, the chapters have been sequenced so that they track the steps usually followed when drafting a medical translation.

We do not envisage medical translation as including only texts for medical specialists. Newspaper reports, advertisements, pharmaceutical and informative leaflets, for instance, are different kinds of texts that deal with or publicize medical discoveries and news, inform patients, persuade international companies to finance a product and so on. As translators, we need to move freely and confidently amongst these and other genres and − if needs be − rewrite the same message for different readers. Therefore, we have also included discussion points and tasks to reflect on and practise these skills.

Finally, we consider the issue of the alleged objectivity and stability of medical language. While it is true that medical language does have many features that tend in this direction, it is also subject to changes and shifts in meaning throughout history, to emotional overtones and to subjective nuances. Exploring the metaphors, the cultural conventions and references, the modulating or hedging techniques sometimes used, the synonyms in the same language, or the lack of equivalence and false friends that exist between languages, reveals gaps in the clarity, precision and conciseness traditionally associated with medical language. The translator often has to deal with "fuzzy edges".

This book has grown out of our professional activity as medical translators, our research and our classroom observation. It includes material and explanations for a 45-60 hour course and is intended for

- Independent learners with a sound awareness of the powers and limitations of language.
- Undergraduate students and teachers in translation and modern languages departments

- Postgraduate students and teachers in translation and modern languages departments
- Professional translators wishing to specialize in the field of medical translation and teaching
- Documentalists working in multilingual medical information management
- Physicians with a professional interest in languages and translation.

Contents and structure

Translation theory will be addressed from a flexible and inductive viewpoint with a special but not exclusive emphasis on the **functionalist** approach as presented by Nord (1997). This approach maintains that when translating it is not only the author or the source text that should be referents, but rather that the translation assignment and the client or the initiator of the translation process are central to the whole decision-making process. The clients or initiators, who could even be the translators themselves, may need the target text to fulfil a different function from that of the source text. This leads us to work with different genres and forms of translation. For example, a client may need a synthetic (summary) translation, or a specialized report to be rewritten as an informative sheet for patients, or research published in specialized journals is often translated for newspaper health supplements adapting the lexis, syntax, register and so on. Therefore, the translator should be loyal to the function or purpose of the assignment, and equivalence, instead of referring to literal translation as has often been held traditionally, becomes a much more flexible concept.

Starting from this broad communication framework that takes into account the differing backgrounds of potential readers, the book basically follows a top-down approach to medical translation: issues of translation and communication > genres > texts > terms and other units of specialized knowledge. Each section will meet the expectations of linguists, translators and medical practitioners in differing degrees. This book is a flexible tool: you can go through it systematically from beginning to end or dip into any part of it in any order according to your needs. It can be used as an accessible introduction to the subject for self-study, or by teachers as a resource book or as a course book that can be complemented with other materials. It is positively focused in that it does not insist on error analysis, but rather on ways of writing good translations and empowering both experts and novices.

Each chapter includes tasks and a section in which a selection of recommended further reading references can be found. The section "Further tasks" at the end of each chapter and the self-study exercises in each chapter are suggestions and starting points that can be adapted to different environments. The tasks for self-study can also be adapted for group practice and the collaborative exercises can be adapted for self-study. A crucial point is that the tasks are not restricted to any two particular languages but can be applied to most language pairs because the emphasis is on learning and on translation transference skills in general – for instance, advice on solving resourcing problems, or the application of appropriate strategies or procedures are relevant to the majority of language contexts.

Full references to the works cited in the book can be found in the bibliography at the end of the book. For ease of use, the sources for sample texts and materials for the different tasks proposed are cited with the texts themselves. Similarly, references for resources and further reading are given in the appropriate chapters and not repeated in the end bibliography.

Translator training in a learner-centred environment

Research in pedagogy and psychology (see, among others, Arnold (ed) 1999; Baer and Koby (eds) 2003; Gardner and Wallace 1972; González Davies 1998, 2004; González Davies and Scott-Tennent 2005; Kiraly 2000; Kussmaul 1995; Nunan 1988, 1989; Richards and Rodgers 1986 / 2001) shows that learning is enhanced when

- it is meaningful to the learners and caters for their needs,
- it takes into account the learners' backgrounds and adapts to their initial level,
- the learners have a say in the proceedings,
- learner autonomy is encouraged,
- a positive and relaxed learning environment is achieved,
- self-confidence is encouraged,
- there is interaction amongst the participants: learners, teachers and, in our case, medical specialists,
- *both* individual and group work are carried out,
- there is space for different kinds of classroom procedures and dynamics to attain the final aims: lectures, pair and group work, learners-learners, teacher-learners and learners-teacher-specialists discussions, and real life (or, if not possible, simulation) assignments,
- authentic, real life activities, tasks and projects can be carried out alongside more pedagogical ones that build on the foundations for a better future professional performance,
- different learning and translating styles are respected.

The emphasis here lies on positive decision-making, problem-spotting and solving with an appropriate application of a wide range of translation strategies and procedures, and the acquisition of linguistic, cognitive, encyclopaedic and professional translation competence.

Our aim in this book is to suggest discussion points and ideas that provide adequate support so that the readers can develop their autonomy and self-confidence alongside the necessary declarative and operative knowledge. We hope to help you with guidelines and tips to justify your translation choices, cooperate with fellow translators, and find what Campbell (1991: 339) describes as a balance between risk-taking and prudence when translating, and between being perseverant or capitulating when under real life constraints such as time, space, money, equipment, faulty originals, difficult clients, and so on.

In other words, we will suggest activities, tasks and projects to help you build on your own previous knowledge and, in the case of a group or classroom setting, that of your peers in a socially positive environment that encourages learner autonomy and the acquisition of self-confidence: an environment in which people are transacting business that is meaningful to them (Kiraly 2000).

1. Introduction to professional practice

> [...] the exponential increase in international communications and the surge of globalization in the business world will lead translators to play a larger and more visible role, and will require increased systematic training of specialized translators.
>
> Françoise Massardier-Kenney (1998)

Overview of chapter

Grasping the relevance of translation through history (1.1) is a way of enhancing self-awareness and identity as a professional translator. Medical translation has some characteristic features that translators should be aware of (1.2). An overview of the working process provides a clearer idea of what happens in a real professional context (1.3). Knowing how the medical translation market works helps translators to find the right professional niche (1.4). Contact with other translators provides insights into how the profession actually works (1.5). To become proficient and competent, we need to acquire and develop certain skills, knowledge and attitudes (1.6). Some tasks (1.7) and suggestions for further reading (1.8) are presented at the end of the chapter.

1.1 Historical overview of medical translation

> Nescire autem quid ante quam natus sis acciderit, id est semper esse puerum.
> [To be ignorant of what occurred before you were born is to remain always a child.]
>
> Marcus Tullius Cicero
> *De optimo genere oratorum*

Translation has probably existed in some form or other ever since human beings felt the need to communicate with other groups of their own kind. Probably the oldest forms of translation involved trade. We find one of the most remote references to written translation in the cities of Ancient Mesopotamia where medical, chemical, mathematical, and astrological knowledge was gathered, organized and stored in cuneiform symbols written on clay tablets, some of which contained information in different languages such as Ugaritic, Akkadian, Sumerian, Hittite, and Hurrian. These archaeological findings suggest an intense translation activity long before paper and the alphabet were invented.

Much later, in the 5th century BCE, Hippocrates – author of one of the oldest volumes on medicine that exist, the *Corpus Hippocraticum*, written about 400

BCE – inherited a vast amount of knowledge from previous civilizations and founded a school of medicine where he produced works on anatomy, physiology, pathology, hygiene, and medical ethics with the collaboration of other scholars. Later, Alexandria, founded by the Greeks in Egypt, became a melting pot for people and ideas, languages and cultures from the Mediterranean lands, the East, and India. We know that its museum and library contained works on anatomical dissections and physiological experiments. Its zoological garden had collections of animals which were classified by scholars and which would have provided opportunities for veterinary research and the study of animal husbandry. Medicinal and other plants in the extensive botanical gardens were similarly classified and their properties were no doubt investigated both for medical and culinary purposes.

A hundred years or so later, the Greek city of Pergamon in Asia Minor became another important centre of scholarship and one which produced Galen, one of the most famous exponents of Greek medical knowledge. He was a prolific author, writing some four hundred works based on the Hippocratic tradition. In the 9th century much of his work was translated into Arabic at the House of Wisdom in Baghdad. These translations, in turn, were translated into Latin in the 11th century, together with commentaries added by other Arab scholars in the intervening years. Thanks to the translation activity carried out at the House of Wisdom, the Arabs assimilated the Greek medical legacy and started to produce original works, which contributed to the advance of medical knowledge.

In Spain, the School of Toledo (1125-52) arose from collaboration between Islamic, Christian, and Jewish scholars. Works by Aristotle (384-322 BCE), Archimedes (287-212 BCE), Pythagoras (569-475 BCE) and Hippocrates (460-377 BCE) were translated and commented upon by physicians such as Ibn-Rushd, also known as Averroes (1126-1198), Maimonides (1135-1204) and Ibn-Sina or Avicenna (980-1037), the author the *Canon Medicinae*, a medical textbook still used in the 18th century. King Alphonse X of Castile (1221-84) introduced translations into Romance Castilian and other emerging European languages at a time when the use of vernacular languages was increasing. In England, King Alfred the Great (871-900), two centuries or so earlier, had promoted education and the arts. He himself translated books from Latin into Anglo-Saxon and ordered translations into that language.

During the Middle Ages knowledge of medicine and related fields was preserved in monastic libraries and medicine was produced and largely dispensed by monks who based many of their medicinal remedies on the accumulated wisdom handed down through the centuries via translations. The continuum of medical knowledge clearly stretches back into pre-historic times.

So far, we have said nothing about how these early works were translated. Were they literal translations? Or were they fairly free and selective adaptations? This dichotomy between strictly literal and freely adapted translations was in fact mentioned by Cicero, whose defence of translating *non verbum de verbo, sed sensum exprimere de sensu* (not word for word, but sense for sense) was expounded in his work *De optimo genere oratorum* (46 BCE). His division has carried over into discussions about translation to the present day. That translation mattered in Ancient Rome is testified to by the fact that the Emperor Augustus employed translators on a regular basis. Medicine was a highly respected discipline at that time and medical translators abounded, working mostly from Greek into Latin. They favoured a literal approach to translation at odds with that of Cicero, whose freer approach was favoured by medieval translators.

In the Middle Ages, this literal view of translation was defended by philosophers and theologians such as Boethius (480-524 AD). Since the Bible was considered to be God's direct revelation to humanity, it was unacceptable to move away from his word towards what might be considered an interpretation. St Jerome's double approach in his Vulgate reflected this dilemma. He defended the classical rhetorical sense for sense approach to translation, but found himself trying to balance it with what he called *veritas*, the truth in the source text, in order to avoid the risk of being accused of heresy.

In the Renaissance, with Latin as the *lingua franca*, two kinds of translations were carried out: between vernacular languages and Latin, and between the vernacular languages themselves. The inclusion of vernacular glosses in Latin translations and the rise of vernacular literatures in the tenth century, together with the invention of printing in the fifteenth century, brought about great changes for translation and its status. Trade and artistic exchanges called for either a *lingua franca* or for a greater emphasis on translation. The growing political importance of vernacular languages, symbolizing the rise of nation states, tipped the scales favourably for translation. Translations of the Bible also represented a milestone in the consolidation of vernacular languages.

The need for a *lingua franca* became acute in the seventeenth century, especially when scientists hoped for a wide distribution of their work. Many translated their works into Latin in order to make them accessible to a wider readership. However, many such works were then plagiarized. Robert Boyle (1627-1691), for instance, was a victim of this type of intellectual theft and finally arranged with the Oxford presses for his works to be published in vernacular English and in Latin simultaneously. Others such as Hobbes (1588-1679) and Newton (1642-1727) followed his example. Most scientists controlled the translations of their work: Descartes' translator was his friend the Duc de Luynes and Newton's was his pupil Samuel Clarke. Translation into Latin on scientific topics died out around 1750.

Two hundred years later, since the middle of the twentieth century, communicative and functional approaches to translation (Reiss and Vermeer 1984/1991, Nord 1997) have made headway in Translation Studies and are especially useful for medical translation. They relate languages to their context and underline the importance of the real world circumstances under which utterances acquire their meaning and should be interpreted, and point out how the translator's choices are conditioned by the client.

The fact that over the last two centuries English has become the new *lingua franca* of distribution does not necessarily mean that it is the only language of production. Biomedical researchers all over the world writing in many different languages try to get their work accepted by international journals published in English through translations. Legal requirements for documentation of medicinal products in the European Union as well as the general trend towards internationalization have also increased the need for translation. In addition, there are bilingual editions of medical journals along with monolingual publications in all languages. Thus, the existence of a *lingua franca* does not necessarily reduce the amount of translation. Most professional translation in the field of medicine or related areas involves English either as a source language or as a target language.

It is difficult to ascertain the actual percentage of medical translations – including all genres, such as research articles, patient information leaflets, advertisements, and so forth – carried out in most countries, but in the case of medical books in Spain, for instance, the information can be easily accessed at the website of the *Ministerio de Cultura* <http://www.mcu.es>. It states that 26% of books published yearly are translations, of which about 10% are medical or scientific.

Task 1. Market research (I)

Find out what the situation in a country of your choice is nowadays as far as medical literature published in translation is concerned: number of yearly publications, percentage of publications which are translations, percentage of translations which are medical texts, legal requirements for documentation of medicinal products, and so forth. Legal and official information from Ministries and other international and national authorities may help.

Knowing something about the history of medical translation and about the differing views on translating that have existed at given historical moments is no frill, for it can help us to understand our position in the professional world better, to be aware of different translation strategies and the functions translations have fulfilled at different stages, to be critical and analytical while considering alternatives, and to learn to justify our choices and argue in an informed way about them. It may also help us to understand better different ways of thinking, writing, and arguing, and to build bridges between scientists, physicians, students, patients, and the general public from different cultures.

The alternative is to work routinely and inflexibly, in a void, with no awareness of the history of the profession. In order to avoid that type of situation most university medical programmes include courses on the History of Medicine. By being aware of our history, translators can become part of this fascinating activity laying to rest once and for all the infamous and untrue *traduttori traditore*, and assuming our true role as active agents in the areas of thought and science.

Task 2. History of medical translation

Find examples of medical translators and translations in your own nation's history: period, branch of knowledge, political context, languages involved, function of the translation, profile of the translator, and other aspects you think are relevant to understand them. Encyclopaedic and academic sources may be helpful. You can read Van Hoof's article 'A contribution to the History of Medical Translation in Japan' (see Further Reading at the end of the chapter) as an example of an introduction to a national history of medical translation.

1.2 The specifics of medical translation

Medical translation shares many features with other types of translation. As in screen, legal or literary translation, it is a professional activity determined by the assignment; it involves adaptation of cultural differences; medical translators also make use of technological tools such as translation memories and electronic dictionaries; their main purpose is also to facilitate communication between different linguistic communities; and so forth. Now, though, let us turn specifically to medical translation and consider what distinguishes it from other types of translation.

Medical specialties

Medical translation involves the communication of knowledge generated and needed in various specialties (see chapter 3) including among many others:

- Internal Medicine: the diagnosis and treatment of cancer, infections, and diseases affecting the heart, blood, kidneys, joints, and digestive, respiratory, and vascular systems; disease prevention, substance abuse, and treatment of problems of the eyes, ears, skin, nervous system, and reproductive organs
- Obstetrics and Gynaecology: the medical and surgical care of the female reproductive system and associated disorders
- Orthopaedics: preservation, investigation, and restoration of the form and function of the extremities, spine, and associated structures; musculoskeletal problems including congenital deformities, trauma, infections, tumours, metabolic disturbances of the musculoskeletal system, deformities, injuries,

and degenerative diseases of the spine, hands, feet, knee, hip, shoulder, and elbow

- Paediatrics: diagnosis and treatment of infections, injuries, genetic defects, malignancies, and many types of organic disease and dysfunction in children
- Psychiatry: prevention, diagnosis, and treatment of mental, addictive, and emotional disorders such as schizophrenia and other psychotic disorders, mood, anxiety, substance-related, sexual and gender identity, and adjustment disorders
- Surgery: preoperative, operative, and postoperative care for a broad spectrum of surgical conditions affecting almost any part of the body
- Pharmacology: drug composition; mechanisms of drug action; therapeutic use of drugs.

When translating medical texts, we may also have to deal with knowledge from anthropology, psychology, sociology, economics and law, among many other disciplines.

Comprehension of medical notions

Factual comprehension is a key element in any translation process, being relevant not only for the translator as a reader of the source text but also for the reader of the target text. However, the priorities are different in medical translation. Whereas the literary translator's main focus is normally on aspects such as register, rhythm, puns, character's attitude, or cultural references, the medical translator's priority is to deal adequately with factual complexity and accuracy. Gaps in the translator's medical knowledge of the different specialties often give rise to comprehension problems. This lack of previous knowledge can be overcome with the help of a range of strategies for acquiring medical knowledge. Wakabayashi's quotation, which opens chapter 3, captures what is essential: a broad understanding of the fundamentals and a knowledge of how to acquire, in the most efficient manner, an understanding of other elements as and when necessary. Chapter 3 focuses on the importance of understanding the contents of the text. Chapter 6 is devoted to acquiring the knowledge needed to be able to understand the source text, to solve translation problems through appropriate resourcing, and to write the target text.

Medical terminology

Terms for anatomical parts, diseases, syndromes, drugs, medical equipment, and so forth are specific to medical translation. Becoming familiar with the particular terminology in the languages involved and being able to solve all sorts of terminological problems – neologisms, synonyms, polysemy, register mismatches – are not only central activities in medical translation but key aspects in the life-long education of professional translators. It should be noted that in the translation process more than half of the time is invested in detecting and solving terminological problems. Chapter 7 deals at length with the basics of medical terminology.

Medical communicative situations

The range of communicative situations where medical translations may be required is very broad, covering not only communication among researchers but also any kind of communicative interaction about health that involves health professionals, patients, and the general public. Among the main communicative functions of medical translation are the following: the dissemination of biomedical research among specialists; the dissemination of the most relevant research in the mass media; the education of health professionals at Universities; the education of patients; the approval of new drugs; the regulation of all kinds of health products; the advertising of health products and services; the communication in hospitals and other health centres; the campaigns carried out by health institutions in the national and international contexts, such as the World Health Organization; and so forth. Medical communicative situations are normally found in the following sectors: biomedical research, health services, pharmaceutical laboratories, publishers in the health sciences, governmental health organizations, non-governmental health organizations, mass media specializing in health matters, and so forth. Chapter 2 focuses on the importance of understanding medical communication.

Medical genres

Thus medical translation covers a wide spectrum of genres: from research articles published in highly specialized journals, to clinical guides for physicians, text books for University students, patient information brochures, press releases, and TV documentaries about health. From a professional point of view, it should be stressed that medical translation is not restricted to highly specialized genres but also includes more general ones. Chapter 2 focuses on genre conventions as one of the key aspects when writing the target text. Chapter 4 deals with target text drafting methodologies in which target genre conventions guide the writing process.

Medical information sources

Professional translators in the health sectors are in constant need of up-to-date sources of medical information of all kinds: explanations of concepts (including pictures, drawings, films and animations); specialized definitions; lists of terms in different languages; nomenclatures; classifications of diseases; lists of drugs with non-proprietary names, trade names and national names; texts belonging to the broad spectrum of medical genres; medical data bases; health directories; online professional forums; information about the clients; information about writing and document style; and so forth. Research for printed, electronic and personal sources is a key feature in medical translation for two reasons: 1) the translator may not have enough factual knowledge to understand the source text, and 2) the translator may have insufficient terminological, and phraseological information as well as inadequate familiarity with target genre conventions to write the target text in an acceptable way. Chapter 6 is fully devoted to medical information sources.

Quality of medical texts

When translating poems, novels, plays or film scripts there is no doubt that the authors of the source texts are skilled writers. The same cannot always be said when dealing with medical texts. More often than not, medical authors are not professional writers. Besides, not all authors of texts about health write in their mother tongue. This means that translators sometimes have to cope with poor quality source texts. There is yet a further consideration: not all source texts received as assignments are finished, ready-to-publish texts. Some are written to be used internally and less care is taken in their finished structure and form while in others authors may implicitly or explicitly rely on translators to revise and edit the source text before writing it in another language. Clearly, then, there are times when translators should not always rely on the quality of the original when taking decisions about the coherence and style of the translation.

Medical ethics

Medical translation is often affected by medical ethics and responsibility. One of the most important ethical norms both in medicine and in medical translation is to act with knowledge and skill since the health or even the lives of patients are often at stake. Hence the critical importance of accuracy and validity of information. Another equally important ethical value in medical translation practice is confidentiality. Medical translators must respect the privacy of patient histories, informed consents, drug development documentation, and medical patents among other genres. Finally medical translators should promote understanding, respect and empathy towards disabled people, towards patients' different sensitivities as far as their diseases are concerned, and towards different cultural views on health and disease. Thus ethical priorities differ in different communicative situations. The following table shows how ethical priorities differ in different genres and demand different skills from the translators:

Genre	Priority
Informed consent	Clarity so that the patient can make a conscious choice.
Original article	Accuracy so that the experiments can be repeated and that the argumentation can be followed in detail.
Patient information leaflet	Clarity so that the patient can take the drug in a safe and effective way.
Questionnaires (evaluation tools)	Cultural relevance so that the questions are meaningful for patients in the target culture.
Clinical history	Confidentiality so as to protect the patient's rights of privacy. Completeness and accuracy so that health professionals in other locations have easy access to the history of the patients. It is also the case that clinical histories can be used as evidence in order to prove clinical negligence of physicians or institutions.
Health campaign	Respect and empathy towards specific groups of patients, disabled people, members of ethnic minorities, etc.

Figure 1.1. Ethical priorities in medical genres

1.3 Steps in the translation process

The aim of this section is to provide an overview of the different steps involved in a typical professional translation process. Each of the steps involves different tasks and requires different skills that you will develop and improve as you get involved in the profession. Although producing the target text is the most visible step, there are other tasks without which the whole process would probably fail, such as analyzing the needs of the client and planning the project. Depending on the assignment, in professional practice medical translators will go through some – mainly the first five and the last one – or all of the following steps.

Analyzing the needs of the client and planning the project

On receiving an assignment, you should discuss the specifics of the project with the client. For information on how to gather all the data you need to start the project, see subsection 'The translation assignment' below. Once you have a firm agreement with your client, you should plan the project: coordination with other translators if necessary, terminology management, contact with experts in the field if necessary, and so forth.

Reading and understanding the source text

It goes without saying that in order to translate a medical text properly, you need to read it thoroughly and have an adequate understanding of it (see chapter 3). Comprehension of particular terms is necessary but of itself is not enough. A broad understanding of the whole text is also required: networks and hierarchies of terms; conceptual links between paragraphs; conceptual links between sections of the same text; descriptive, narrative and argumentative structures; overall cause and effect relationships. If you don't have enough background information to understand your source text, you should try reading less specialized texts about the same topic and get immersed in it gradually.

Compiling a glossary

Glossaries are used to ensure that terminology is consistent 1) internally with the solutions adopted in a particular assignment, and 2) externally with the client's norms and preferences. In addition, compiling our own dictionary will allow us to acquire new concepts by means of definitions and to better understand conceptual relationships between different terms. Glossary compilation should be done in such a way as to allow us to retrieve and use those terms and definitions again in the future or to share them online with other translators. Hence the convenience of using electronic terminology managers. See chapter 7 for more on terminology.

Drafting the target text

Once you have understood the source text and have compiled the glossary, you are in a comfortable and self-confident position to start drafting the target text (see chapter 4), be it a full translation, a summarized adaptation or whatever the client needs. In the first draft it is important to focus attention on the two most basic aspects of text production: structure and contents. We must consider both the macro structure of the target text − sections, subsections, moves, flow of information, etc., which may or may not coincide with that of the source text − and the factual information the structure should contain. It is like digging the foundations, and erecting the pillars that will support all the other parts of the building. Our aim now is accuracy in bringing to the target text at least the most relevant information contained in the source text and putting it in the right place. We will also deal with most translation problems at this point (chapter 5).

Conceptual and formal details will be sorted out later in further drafts in which we will focus on micro-elements such as links between sentences, word order, terminological choices, etc.

Revising and editing the target text

Once structure and factual information are in place, then we can start revising and editing for conceptual completeness, accuracy, clarity, cohesion, syntax, in-house style, grammar, spelling, punctuation and consistency in the use of terms, abbreviations, numbers, proper names, etc. When revising and editing it is important to follow a logical sequence of steps starting from contents and ending in spelling and punctuation (see chapter 4).

Proofreading

Once you have revised and edited the target text – against the source text and on its own – through different drafts then you can produce a document that should read as an autonomous, finished text. When proofreading we make sure that the text reads well, paying special attention to punctuation, spelling, quantities, numerical expressions, and so forth.

Reviewing the translation by the client

Sometimes clients may revise the finished translation before it is formatted and printed for publication. Their comments are often valuable and can help us to meet their needs.

Formatting

Once the text has been fully accepted by the client it can be formatted in the required format: Page Maker, QuarkXPress, HTML, PDF and other. The translator is normally expected to be fully conversant with these and other tools.

Reviewing the galley

Galley review is carried out when the target text is to be printed and published. Depending on the publisher and/or printer, galley review is carried out either internally as one more step of book production or it is commissioned to the translators. In galley review correct hyphenation, font size, font type, page numbering, and footnote numbering, are revised. Sometimes galleys are also reviewed by clients to ensure that not only the text but also the document will meet their needs.

Delivering the final document to the client

Finally the document is produced and delivered to the client in the form agreed: e-mail, FTP, or CD sent by ordinary post.

In the rest of the chapters we will look in greater detail at the most basic steps presented so far: analyzing the needs of your client as far as readership is concerned (chapter 2), reading and understanding the source text (chapters 2, 3 and 6), solving translation problems (chapter 5), compiling a glossary (chapters 3, 6 and 7), and drafting and revising the target text (chapters 4 and 5).

1.4 Approaching the market

In the era of the Internet and globalization, the translation market we can aim at is no longer restricted to our place of residence. Working online for clients and other translators we never meet in person is fast becoming the norm. Another important feature of the translation market is its dynamism: it changes in tandem with new scientific and technological developments as well as with new communication needs. In this section you will find some basic information about types of clients, types of tasks and most frequently translated genres, which should help to give you some direction in your professional development.

Types of clients

Clients fall into two main groups: those in the public sector and those in the private one.

Public sector

- International institutions such as the *European Commission* translation services
  <http://www.europa.eu.int>, the *Red Cross* <http://www.icrc.org>, the *World Health Organization*, the *Organización Panamericana de Salud*, and other UN bodies. You can have access to job offer in UN organizations at
  <http://www.un.org/Depts/OHRM/>
- Government agencies
- Universities
- Research institutes
- Special attention should be paid to the growing needs for translators in hospitals and health services in general in countries where there is a large immigrant population.

Private sector

- Pharmaceutical laboratories
- Publishers in the health sector
- Private hospitals
- Manufacturers of medical appliances
- Medical software industry
- Private biomedical research centres
- Biotechnology companies
- Health and care managers and professionals

When working for translation agencies the contact with the final client may sometimes be a problem. You can find further information on the European translation market at <http://www.europa.eu.int/eures/index.jsp>.

Common tasks of the medical translator

The skills that translators develop in the course of their work equip them for a wide range of professional opportunities from writing to managing multilingual medical information. In fact, clients frequently ask medical translators to carry out a variety of tasks which may include:

- Translating texts both for internal use and for publication
- Rewriting and adapting texts
- Writing original texts from given information
- Translating and updating web pages of medical content
- Translating medical software
- Translating research articles into English
- Revising and editing translations
- Revising and editing originals
- Revising and editing translation memories
- Creating terminological data bases of medical terms
- Finding and organizing medical information in multilingual contexts
- Translating and adapting medical dictionaries of health topics
- Planning and managing translation projects
- Interpreting in hospitals and other health services

To interpret at medical conferences you need special training in conference interpreting techniques. However, key issues in medical translation such as the acquisition of background knowledge, the comprehension of medical notions, terminology management and effective use of sources of medical information dealt with in this chapter are also extremely relevant to the practice of conference interpreting.

As the above list shows, medical translators do not simply translate. They have also become writers, terminologists, revisers, web creators, multilingual knowledge managers, language quality control experts, community interpreters, and communication experts.

The translation assignment

The assignment is both the starting point and the goal of any professional translation process. Translators should be loyal not only to the contents of the source text but also to the translation assignment as described by the client. This approach to translation was forefronted and widely discussed when Katarina Reiss and Hans Vermeer published *Grundlegung einer allgemeinen Translationstheorie* (1984). Their work brought about a dramatic breakthrough in Translation Studies mainly because they were the first to suggest that the *skopos* or function of a text is the translator's main concern. This challenges the traditional view that the author or the text are the starting points of a translation. Christiane Nord took this further in her books *Text Analysis in Translation* (1988/1991) and *Translating as a Purposeful Activity* (1997) where she presented a translation theory that aimed at reconciling academic and professional viewpoints and interests: functionalism. At its core is that the translator should be loyal only to the translation *assignment* as described by its *initiator* (or client). Thus, the translator has to perform according to Lasswell's well-known key question when talking about communication (1948 in Nord 1991): "Who says what in which channel to whom with what effect?". Reiss, Vermeer and Nord have taken this further and included additional questions such as: "when, where, why and how?". So, the final target text will depend on the function of the translation as given by its initiator when defining the assignment. It follows that different degrees of fidelity will have to be applied according to the translation assignment (e.g. the "translation" of a specialized text for the medical section of a newspaper). This may require a change of style, register, lexis, or syntax. These adjustments are directly related both to the nature of translation and to the wide range of what we call "medical" texts: from original articles, reviews, case studies, or editorials to pharmaceutical leaflets, ads, journalistic rewriting, medical language in advertising, literature or drama and so on. Translators will need to be familiar with all these text types (seee chapter 2). When specifying the translation assignment a number of important points should be considered, such as:

- What product or service does the client need? (See subsection 'Common tasks of the medical translator' above).
- What is the profile of the target audience? (See section 'Participants in

medical communication and their purposes' in Chapter 2)
- In which context and communicative situations will the target text be used?
- What is the purpose of the target text? (See section 'Participants in medical communication' and their purposes in Chapter 2)
- What is the profile of the organization that will use the target text? Are there in-house style norms?
- Are there legal requirements that may affect the production of the target text?
- Does the client or organization that will use the translation have terminological preferences?
- Does the client have terminological glossaries and/or other documentation that may be helpful for us?
- Which format of delivery is required?
- What is the deadline for delivery?

It is the translator's responsibility to find out all necessary information as far as the assignment is concerned, even if the client does not provide it straight away. Clients are not always aware of the information translators need before they undertake a given project. Last, but not least, it is always advisable to provide an estimate of the cost of any work to be carried out.

Task 3. Exploring the *skopos* (purpose) of assignments

Imagine a real assignment. For instance, you have been asked to translate medical research that has been published in a prestigious professional journal for the Health Section of a mainstream newspaper. Answer the following general questions to analyze the communicative situation of both source texts and target texts of this kind:

- Who says
- what,
- when,
- where,
- why,
- how,
- to whom and
- to what effect?

Frequently translated genres

In this section some of the most frequently translated genres are presented so that you have a clearer idea of the variety of text forms with which medical translators deal (see 2.5 for a more detailed description of them). For ease of use, these genres have been divided into four categories according to their main roles in society: research, professional practice, education and trade. Some of them, however, can be included in more than one category. This is the case, for example, of dictionaries, encyclopaedias, web pages, and summaries of product characteristics, the function of which is to inform the physician about a particular drug so that it can be safely prescribed and, therefore, sold by the laboratory.

Research genres are the genres used by researchers and physicians working in hospitals, research centres, laboratories and universities in any medical speciality to communicate their findings and arguments. They are sources of primary information – new information that has not been published before. Most of them are highly standardized.

- Research papers (see chapter 4)
- Review articles (see chapter 2)
- Clinical trial protocols (see chapter 2)
- Case reports (see chapter 2)
- Metaanalyses
- Short communications
- Letters to the editor
- Scientific editorials
- Position papers
- Book reviews
- Conference proceedings
- Doctoral theses

Professional genres are used by health professionals – doctors, nurses, technicians, and managers – in the course of their work in clinics and in the health industry. Typical genres in this category are:

- Clinical guidelines (see chapter 2)
- Standard operating procedures (see chapter 2)
- Summary of product characteristics (see chapter 2)
- Informed consents (see chapter 2)
- Lab tests
- Medical questionnaires
- Medical terminology glossaries
- Manuals
- Maintenance guides
- Annual reports
- Bulletins

- Expert reports
- Medical histories
- Disease classifications
- Nomenclatures
- Medical dictionaries
- Vademecums
- Software interfaces

Educational genres are used to teach and learn in a wide range of contexts, from university courses to institutional campaigns to domestic life.

- Fact sheets for patients (see chapter 2)
- Patient information leaflets (see chapter 2)
- Course books
- Treatises
- Training courses
- Presentations
- Popularizing articles
- Medical encyclopaedias
- Summaries for patients
- TV documentary scripts

Commercial genres are used to sell and buy products and services of all kinds in the health sectors.

- Drug advertisements (see chapter 2)
- Contracts
- Vial and carton labels
- Product information leaflets
- Catalogues
- New drug applications
- Packaging inserts
- Patents
- Press releases

1.5 Socializing with peers

Translation is often a lonely activity and we can easily feel isolated or in need of support and reassurance from others who understand our difficulties and who are willing to share their ideas and expertise. Nowadays such help is available from groups of translators who have lively exchanges and debates on the Internet.

These groups may be organized in a variety of ways and may differ in orientation, interests and styles of communication. Some are hierarchical and formal – you may only join if invited to do so and you may have to submit a CV – whereas others are informal and open to all. Some have a very restricted view of translation and focus almost entirely on terminological problems, while others take a much broader view and include matters of culture and communication. And, of course, although all of us are aware of the importance of cultural differences when translating, we musn't forget this when we communicate with other translators whose cultural norms may differ from our own. Exploring and understanding the following aspects will help you decide which is the best group for you and become one its members:

- How do they communicate with each other? (distribution lists, forums, etc.)
- What kind of language (formal, chatty, etc.) do they use?
- What metalanguage about translation do they use?
- What publications do they read?
- What kinds of information do they exchange?
- What translation resources do they use?
- What types of assignments do they receive?
- What do existing members appear to expect from new ones?

The second step is becoming an accepted and active member of that community while, at the same time, retaining your own independence and individuality. Through discussing and exchanging all kinds of information – about fees, job offers, working methods, new tools, sources of information, translation problems and solutions, etc. – with other professional translators you will gain insight into how your profession works and will be able to find your own niche within it. Reading translators' journals and bulletins, and participating in meetings, online forums, distribution lists, and courses will be useful in this respect. Life-long education of the medical translator is essential for a successful career.

Task 4. Professional practice (I)

1) Choose one of the professional associations – ideally one related to your own circumstances.
2) Explore the site you have chosen and find out information about:

- Fees
- Advertising facilities for freelance translators
- Contact with clients
- Professional accreditation

- Legal rights
- Ethical codes
- Membership: how to become a member, advantages, etc.
- Continuing education programmes
- Forums, chats, distribution lists
- Bulletins, journals of the professional associations
- Sections devoted to medical translation or to scientific and techn-cal translation
- Recommended links
- Professional associations.

Professional associations

- Medicina y traducción (Medtrad)
- International Federation of Translators
- Society for Technical Communication
- European Medical Writers Association
- American Medical Writers Association
- Australian Medical Writers Association
- World Association of Science Editors
- Council of Science Editors
- Society of Medical Interpreters
- American Translators Association
- Institute of Translation and Interpreting
- Assoziierte Dolmetscher und Übersetzer
- Société Française des Traducteurs
- Austrian Translators and Interpreters Association
- Associació de traductors i intèrprets de Catalunya
- Traductors i intèrprets associats pro-col•legi
- Asociación española de traductores, correctores e intérpretes
- Association professionnelle des métiers de la traduction
- Finnish Association of Translators and Interpreters
- Swiss Association of Translators, Terminologists and Interpreters
- Union of Interpreters and Translators (Czech and Slovak Republics)
- Norwegian Non-Fiction Writers and Translators Association
- The Swedish Association of Professional Translators
- Union of Translators of Russia
- Japan Association of Translators
- South African Translator's Institute
- Australian Institute of Interpreters and Translators Incorporated
- New Zealand Society of Translators and Interpreters
- Asociación Argentina de Traductores e Intérpretes
- Associação Brasiliense de Traductores e Intérpretes

- Asociación de traductores e intérpretes de Monterey
- Asociación de traductores profesionales de Perú
- Asociación Mexicana de traductores
- Massachusetts Medical Interpreters Association
- Irish Translators' and Interpreters' Association

Task 5. Professional associations

1) Choose another professional association unconnected with your geographical environment.
2) Compare the information it provides with what you discovered in the
   previous task.

- What are the main differences between the associations you have explored in the previous task and the ones you have chosen for this one?
- Is there any organizational or professional aspect that you think associations relevant to your environment might consider adopting? Which?
  Explain why.

1.6 Becoming a medical translator: specific competencies

Drawing on the specifics of medical translation, on the stages of the translation
process in a professional context and on the medical translation market, in this
section we present a selection of the competencies that may help you to become
a professional medical translator either through self-study or following specialized courses or both. Before we go into competencies, however, we would like
to touch on a common debate among translators, teachers, and students, that is,
who should translate medical texts.

Are doctors the only people that can translate medical texts well? Not necessarily. Can doctors who translate be sensitive enough to linguistic and cultural
issues to become good medical translators? Yes, they can. According to Fernando
Navarro, a leading medical translator with a medical degree,

> Today, specialisation has become a requirement for translators and many
> other professionals – amongst them, doctors. It is professional translators
> who specialise in medical texts – whether they come from the world of
> medicine, translation or any other discipline – whom I would consider as
> 'medical translators' (in Márquez, 2000).

Marla O'Neill (1998: 80) goes a step further:

> Good medical translation can be done by both medical professionals
> and medically knowledgeable linguists; but in both cases (Woody Allen
> notwithstanding), a love for language, an ear for style, a willingness to
> pursue arcane terminology, and caring enough to get it exactly right are
> the keys to true success.

And linguists with appropriate medical knowledge can also produce good medical translations as well.

A distinction can be made between comprehension, on the one hand, and knowledge and skill, on the other. Take this example: to understand and explain a cataract operation you don't need to be an ophthalmologist. Comprehending the cataract operation is necessary but not enough to perform it: one needs to know how to do it, and not just to understand how it is done by others. What medical translators need is to comprehend the cataract operation, not to be able to perform it. Comprehension takes place at a basic level in the cognition process; knowledge and expertise go beyond understanding and are of a higher order. Hence translators without a medical background can acquire an adequate grasp of a medical subject if they have access to appropriate documentation and develop strategies that enable them to think logically.

As for doctors who have not been trained in linguistic and cultural issues, with appropriate training they can develop adequate writing skills. What matters at this point is not whether the medical translator has a degree in Medicine or Translation, but whether s/he has the translation skills required to be an efficient mediator. So, it is important to concentrate on those skills, regardless of the educational background. As will be seen when exploring translation competence, doctors will be better prepared in some aspects, whereas linguists will be so in others.

Task 6. Mind Maps: What is medical translation?

An eye-opening introductory activity to help you explore issues related to medical translation and bring to the surface your passive knowledge on the subject is to draw a Mind Map reflecting your ideas on medical translation. A Mind Map is a diagram that depicts ideas and concepts, terminology, etc in a personal, flexible and clear way.

Write "Medical Translation" on a big sheet of paper, in the centre of the page, and draw lines that lead to related topics. Each subdivision can then include words, expressions, and other concepts, which may be expanded as you acquire experience in medical translation.

Translation competence refers to the ability, skill or knowledge – both operative (know how) and declarative (know what) − translators need to work in an efficient and professional manner. There is still no agreement on which elements are needed to draw the complete map of translation competence, but in the specific case of medical translators special attention should be paid to the competencies listed below. Although this is not a complete list, it reflects the main areas on which you can focus your gradual, life-long education as a medical translator. For ease of comprehension, the competencies are grouped under the following labels: language and writing; communication and culture; medical notions; transference; information resources; professional practice; and attitude.

Language and writing

You need to be familiar with:
- The most translated genres, especially in the target language, and the formal differences between them
- The form and function of medical terms in the languages involved and the differences between them
- The chemical, generic and trade names of drugs
- Terminological standardization: international nomenclatures, classifications, taxonomies, and so forth
- Medical metaphors and images
- Medical acronyms, abbreviations and symbols
- Medical phraseology especially in the target language
- Linguistic varieties within the same language (e.g. British, American, and Australian English; Castilian, Mexican and Argentinian Spanish, etc.; or Brazilian and Peninsular Portuguese).

You need to know:
- The genre conventions in the languages involved, especially those that may differ between languages
- The Greek and Latin roots, prefixes and suffixes relevant to the formation of medical terminology
- The interferences that can arise between languages, mainly false friends and calques
- The importance of making inferences from textual and contextual elements when trying to understand the source text.

You need to be able to:
- Understand and write original texts belonging to the most translated genres
- Apply in-house style norms so that specific publishers accept the target text
- Deal correctly with terminological variation, in particular that caused by polysemy, synonyms, and homonymous terms

- Apply sound criteria and be creative in supplying medical neologisms in the target language when necessary
- De-terminologize medical terms (turn medical terms into short explanations) in the target text so as to make them comprehensible to lay readers when necessary
- Recognize registers (e.g. palpitations vs tachycardia) and register mismatches between languages
- Pronounce medical terms correctly
- Neutralize the language in order to avoid geographical variations and make the target text readable in any location of the same language.

Task 7. From notes to text

Find an abstract and introduction to a medical article and rewrite it in note form following the procedures below:
1) Read the text and underline key words and phrases
2) Make comments in the margin if necessary
3) Use symbols, acronyms, abbreviations, etc
4) Make the internal structure and the relation between the contents visible by means of
5) Means of symbols such as arrows, mathematical signs, etc.
6) To understand the text fully, read each sentence and reorganise or say it in a different way in your mind.

Reconstruct the introduction from the notes in full text form. Wait a couple of days before trying to rewrite the text.

Compare the text you have written with the original one. For them to co-incide would be quite impossible, but the same message, tone and register should have been kept.

Finally, translate the introduction for a similar publication in another language and correct the translation with the help of parallel texts, resources materials, or other translators and field specialists, if possible.

Communication and culture

You need to be familiar with:
- Different types of target readers, their motivations, their expectations and their purposes in written medical communication, and be able to facilitate their understanding the contents of the source

- Different knowledge communities and their implicit and explicit norms: patients, relatives, physicians, nurses, researchers, managers, technicians, and so forth
- Different types of authors, their working contexts, their motivations and their reasons for writing
- The national health systems pertinent to your translation assignments
- International health organizations such as the World Health Organization.

You need to know:
- Different types of publications and their in-house style norms
- The specific situations in which source and target texts are used
- The legal norms imposed either on the source text or on the target text
- The ethical norms that govern either the source text or the target text
- The differences about the social values and beliefs attached to health and disease in different countries and cultures
- The euphemisms referring to body parts and functions, and the differences in the languages involved.

Task 8. Comparing text types

Read the two texts below. They are on the same topic, but written for a different kind of reader. Spot and underline the stylistic, lexical and text type elements that signal the degree of specialization. Different colours can be used to underline the different stylistic characteristics, for instance, use of nouns, adjectives, verbs or adverbs; medical terminology; impersonal address; idiomatic expressions; humour; historical references; or syntax.

Text A
Scientific Conference Extols New Wonder Drug: Red Wine
By Jennifer Warner

The Daily Telegraph
Oct. 27, 2003

Bordeaux, France — Red wine could inspire new ways to treat AIDS, sleeping sickness, heart disease and cancer, and even to rejuvenate blood and skin, scientists said.

Those were some of the startling findings presented this week at the first symposium on blood and wine, held at Universite Victor Segalen in Bordeaux — the heart of France's most famous wine district.

Scientists have long puzzled over the "French Paradox:" French people suffer less cancer and heart disease than other Europeans, despite a lifestyle long on rich foods and short on exercise. Alcohol is known to increase the risk of harmful clotting. But Prof Serg Renaud of the host university said that this effect was absent in red wine, probably because it contained polyphenols, found in the skins and seeds of grapes.

Prof. Ludovic Drouet of the Hospital Lariboisiere in Paris said studies suggested that wine had a subtle effect on high cholesterol, cell proliferation and blood clotting. At Chateau Smith Haut Lafitte, Bordeaux, where the Cathiard family make fine wines, a process developed by Prof. Joseph Vercauteren is now in use to extract the cocktail for skin products — centuries after Marie Antoinette washed her face in wine to protect against wrinkles.

Dr Marie-Claude Garel of ICGM Maternite de Port-Royal, Paris, told the meeting that a group of polyphenols called resveratrols could reactivate the manufacture of fetal blood in the body. Another researcher said polyphenols could augment conventional AIDS treatments. Resveratrol also possesses anti-cancer properties, said Dr Francis Raul of Strasbourg. But Prof. Djavad Mossalayi of UVS has tested it on human cells, both normal and cancerous, and found it to be toxic to both.

Text B

Am J Clin Nutr. 2003 Aug; 78(2): 334-8

Relation between homocysteine concentrations and the consumption of different types of alcoholic beverages: the French Supplementation with Antioxidant Vitamins and Minerals Study.

Mennen LI, de Courcy GP, Guilland JC, Ducros V, Zarebska M, Bertrais S, Favier A, Hercberg S, Galan P.

UMR INSERM unit 557/INRA unit 1125, Institut Scientifique et Technique de la Nutrition et de l'Alimentation, Paris, France. s_mennen@vcnam.cnam.fr

BACKGROUND: Previous studies on the effects of alcohol consumption on total plasma homocysteine (tHcy) concentrations showed contradictory results. The conflicting results may derive in part from confounding by the type of alcoholic beverage consumed. OBJECTIVE: The objective of the study was to evaluate in a predominantly wine drinking French population whether the relation between alcohol consumption and homocysteine concentrations is dependent on the type of alcoholic beverage consumed. DESIGN: In 1996, a cross-sectional study measuring tHcy and red blood cell folate concentrations was conducted in 1196 middle-aged women and men from the French Supplementation with Antioxidant Vitamins and Minerals Study. Intakes of alcohol, energy, coffee, and B vitamins were assessed by 6 separate 24-h dietary records from the previous year. RESULTS: tHcy concentrations were positively associated with wine intake ($P = 0.01$) in the women and with beer intake in the men ($P = 0.002$). No association with the consumption of spirits was observed. The association between beer consumption and tHcy concentrations in the men was modified by the consumption of wine; the association was positive in wine drinkers, whereas an inverse trend was seen in those who drank no wine. CONCLUSION: Wine consumption may increase tHcy concentrations, whereas beer consumption seems to have no effect (or even an inverse effect) on tHcy.

Medical notions

You need to understand:
- Greek and Latin roots, prefixes and suffixes used in medical terminology
- Main anatomical notions
- Main physiological notions
- Main histological notions
- The mechanisms of main diseases: aetiology, evolution, signs, symptoms, and treatment
- The mechanisms of drugs, their composition, their therapeutic effects and their adverse effects
- Basic statistics and how they are used in biomedical research papers
- The main notions of biochemistry
- The main notions of molecular biology
- The main notions of mental health
- The main notions of public health
- The main instruments used in medicine
- The main tests used in medicine.

Transference

You need to be able to:
- Make sure that the transference process does not alter the facts in the slightest detail
- Make sure that the sense is properly transferred

- Make sure that the information in the target text is true and coherent internally
- Translate across genres, that is, translations in which the target text does not belong to the same genre as the source text
- Introduce conventions from the target genre in the target text
- Carry out self and peer evaluation
- Adapt to appropriate cultural shifts.

You need to know:
- The stages translators go through during the translation process
- Translation strategies and procedures
- The main transference errors in medical translation in order both to anticipate them and avoid them, and to spot problems and correct them.

Task 9. Sight translation of medical texts

Sight translation is is a frequent activity for professional translators. It consists in "reading" a text in a different language from that in which it is written. That is, the translator carries out an oral translation at reading speed without having prepared the translation previously.

This activity will help you spot and solve translation problems quickly, practise speed translation, and develop your translation competence.

Choose a text on a relevant medical topic for which you have a translation available. Translate the text orally and record yourself doing it. Do not look at the published translation. Without stopping, underline any interesting problems that crop up. Finally, listen to yourself and compare your sight translation to the written translation.

Information resources

You need to be able to:
- Find all kinds of medical information: terminological, stylistic, textual, etc.
- Efficiently use medical dictionaries, encyclopaedias, atlases, etc.
- Efficiently use major medical information databases such as Medline
- Evaluate the quality of medical information sources
- Obtain the collaboration of a subject field expert in the translation process when necessary.

You need to know:

- The main organizations that generate and distribute medical information:

book publishers, research journals, international organizations, governmental agencies, non-governmental organizations, mass media, etc.
- The advanced search features of main search engines
- The main terminological data bases.

Professional practice

You need to be able to:
- Carry out market research
- Use specific translation tools
- Negotiate terminological solutions with the clients
- Obtain all kinds of relevant information from the clients
- Communicate fluently with the clients
- Keep to deadlines
- Work in teams.

You need to know:
- Legal issues that may affect medical translation practice
- Fees appropriate for the work you undertake

Task 10. Market research (II)

Here you have the URLs for some of the best-known translation companies working in the biomedical sectors (updated on Google, May 2006). Explore them and find out about:

- Translators' qualifications: required degrees, experience, skills, etc.
- Fees: per word, per page, per hour, per project, etc.
- Quality control systems: technical revision, stylistic revision, etc.
- Translation process: steps, team organization, etc.
- Terminology management: IT, assessment, etc.
- Clients: types of organizations, economic sectors, countries, etc.
- Ideas about translation: what they consider to be a good translation, why, etc.
- Languages: most common combinations, etc.
- Tasks: translating, rewriting, writing, revising, managing projects, terminology compilation, etc.
- Method for recruiting of new translators: exams, interviews, etc...

Translation companies

- *1-800-Translate* <http://www.1-800-translate.com/Medical.html>

- *Applied language solutions*
  <http://www.appliedlanguage.com/medical_translation.shtml>
- *Translators specializing in medicine / medical equipment*
  <http://medizin.li/medical-translation/>
- *Biomedical Translations* <http://www.biomedical.com/>
- *Translation Perfect*
  <http://www.transperfect.com/tp/eng/industry_pharmaceutical.html>
- *Global link translations*
  <http://www.globalinktranslations.com/index.asp>
- Alba Lux <http://www.alba-lux.com/>
- *Lengua Translations*
  <http://www.lengua.com/medical-translation.shtml>
- *Word Lingo*
  <http://www.worldlingo.com/en/solutions/medical_translation.html>
- *Welocalize* <http://www.welocalize.com/english/industries/medical.
  html>
- *RIC International* <http://www.ricintl.com/>
- *Linguistic Systems Inc. Medical Translation Center*
  <http://www.linguist.com/mtc.htm>
- *Excel Translations Inc.* <http://www.xltrans.com/ser_med.html>
- *Trusted Translations* <http://www.trustedtranslations.com/span-
  ish_medical_translation.asp>
- *Enlaso*
  <http://www.translate.com/services/medical_translation.html>
- *Gamax* <http://loc.gamax.hu/med-translation-en.html>
- *RWS Group*
  < http://www.rws-group.com/lang_english/startpage.html >
- *All Language Alliance* <http://www.languagealliance.com/translation-
  services/>
- *Nettprofile* <http://www.nettranslation.co.uk/medical_translation_serv-
  ice.htm>
- *Translation Services USA*
  <http://www.translation-services-usa.com/medical.shtml>
- *Web Translations* <http://www.web-translations.co.uk/EN/Solutions/
  industry/medical.html>
- *Global language solutions* <http://www.globallanguages.com>

Attitude

You need to be able to:
- Understand the full sense of what you do
- Constantly update knowledge about medical translation practice (new market

developments, working tools, subject matter, etc.) and about translation stud-
ies (new research that may improve translation practice)
- Motivate yourself and constantly improve self-concept
- Improve intra- and interpersonal intelligences: balancing risk-taking and
  prudence, and being perseverant or capitulating
- Justify your translation decisions and accept suggestions
- Empathize with peers and clients.

You need to be aware of:
- Your professional identity, especially when working in contexts dominated
  by health professionals
- Your power to change what you don't like about what you do as a professional
  translator
- How subjectivity may influence relationships with peers and clients
- Your strong and weak points as a professional translator
- The importance of developing memory, mental agility and flexibility.

1.7 Further tasks

Task 11. Grasping the relevance of medical translation through history

1) Read the introductory text "Medieval Islam" about medicine and Islamic
   cultures written by Savage-Smith (2001) and published by the National
   Library of Medicine of the United States at <http://www.nlm.nih.gov/hmd/
   arabic/med_islam.html>.
2) Explain why translation has been important in the development of medicine
   through history.

Task 12. Exploring genres

1) Find examples of the genres listed in the section 1.4 under 'Most frequently
   translated genres' in your mother tongue.
2) Tryto explain in which respects knowing about them could be useful in the
   translation process.

1.8 Further reading

Delisle, Jean and Judith Woodsworth (1993) *Translators through History*, Amsterdam
    and Philadelphia: John Benjamins.
Fischbach, Henry (1993) 'Translation, the great pollinator of science: A brief flashback

on Medical Translation', in Sue Ellen Wright and Leland Wright (eds) *Scientific and Technical Translation*, Amsterdam and Philadelphia: John Benjamins, 89-100.

Fischbach, Henry (ed.) (1998) *Translation and Medicine,* Amsterdam and Philadelphia: John Benjamins. [American Translators Association Monographs].

González Davies, Maria (2004) *Multiple Voices in the Translation Classroom. Activities, Tasks and Projects*, Amsterdam and Philadelphia: John Benjamins.

Gutiérrez, Bertha (1998) *La ciencia empieza en la palabra. Análisis e historia del lenguaje científico*, Barcelona: Península.

Lee-Jahnke, Hannelore (1998) 'Training in Medical Translation with Emphasis on German', in Henry Fischbach (ed.) *Translation and Medicine*, Amsterdam and Philadelphia: John Benjamins, 81-92.

------ (2005) 'Teaching medical translation: an easy job?', *Panace@ Revista de Medicina y Traducción* 6(20): 81-84. [Available at: http://www.medtrad.org/panacea]

Márquez, Cristina (2000) 'Entrevista a Fernando Navarro', *Infórmate, Journal of the Spanish of the ATA*, http://www.ata-spd.org/Informate/Entrevistas/fernando_navarro.htm.

Montalt, Vicent (2005) *Manual de traducció cientificotècnica,*in Biblioteca de Traducció i Interpretació, Vic: Eumo.

Montgomery, Scott L. (2000) *Science in Translation. Movements of Knowledge through Cultures and Times*, Chicago and London: The University of Chicago Press.

McMorrow, Leon (1998) 'Breaking the Greco-Roman Mold in Medical Writing: The Many Languages of the 20th Century Medicine', in Henry Fischbach (ed.) *Translation and Medicine*, Amsterdam and Philadelphia: John Benjamins, 13-28.

O'Neill, Marla (1998) 'Who Makes a Better Medical Translator: The Medically Knowledgeable Linguist or the Linguistically Knowledgeable Medical Professional? A Physician's Perspective', in Henry Fischbach (ed.) *Translation and Medicine*, Amsterdam and Philadelphia: John Benjamins, 69-80.

Van Hoof, Henri (1998) 'A contribution to the History of Medical Translation in Japan', in Henry Fischbach (ed.) *Translation and Medicine*, Amsterdam and Philadelphia: John Benjamins, 29-36.

Vickery, Brian (2000) *Scientific Communication in History*, London: The Scarecrow Press.

Wakabayashi, Judith (1996) 'Teaching Medical Translation', *Meta* 41(3): 356-365

Wright, Sue Ellen and Leland Wright (eds) (1993) *Scientific and Technical Translation,* Amsterdam and Philadelphia: John Benjamins. [ATA Scholarly Monograph Series].

2. Understanding medical communication

> Written scientific communication appears then as a multidimensional network of restrained or expanded groups which communicate amongst themselves and, increasingly, with the exterior by means of vulgarization. The resulting discourses are different depending on whether they circulate inside a restrained group where everybody knows each other and shares the same key information, or in larger groups, within the same speciality, or in even wider groups that relate to different specialities. When the key information is not shared entirely, the discourse has to be made more explicit.
>
> O. Régent (1992: 66, in Balliu 2001: 93)

Overview of chapter

Translators are communicators and medical translation is a specific type of medical communication, which like all translation involves different languages and cultures. In this chapter we explore the dynamic nature and wide scope of medical communication (2.1), which is not limited to the interaction among researchers in the biomedical field, but includes health professionals, patients, and the general public. Then we focus on the participants and their communicative purposes (2.2); these are two of the main factors that determine the writing of the source and target texts: different participants with different purposes require different forms of text – we will call them text genres or simply genres. In order to understand written medical communication better, knowledge of the relationships between texts may be useful (2.3). Texts that share the same communicative purpose and that are addressed to the same type of readership normally belong to the same genre (2.4) and, therefore, share formal conventions – such as structure, length, tenor, style, terminology or phraseology. Ten genres common in medical communication and in medical translation will be explored (2.5). Some tasks (2.6) and suggestions for further reading (2.7) are presented at the end of the chapter.

2.1 The dynamic and varied nature of medical communication

Medical communication is not limited to written interaction among researchers in highly specialized research journals. Rather it can be seen as a rich, dynamic continuum moving from research articles to educational television documentaries on relevant health topics or news in the press about health and medicine. In fact, medical knowledge is generated by a variety of participants: researchers, physicians, surgeons, nurses, carers, patients, patients' family members, health managers, health policy makers, medical teachers, medical students, and so forth. Furthermore, medical knowledge may be presented in many different ways: formal or informal, specialized or popular, oral or written. Becoming aware of the dynamism and complexity of medical communication is a key element for a successful career as a medical translator.

Top-down *and* bottom-up

Medical research is conducted as a response to several types of needs: pharmaceutical companies wishing to commercialize new drugs; health authorities wishing to find solutions to general health problems; physicians and patients wishing to improve the treatment of diseases; and so forth. New knowledge is generated by researchers in laboratories and hospitals, and then distributed top-down so that it can benefit patients, companies and the general public.

However, medical knowledge is also generated bottom up. Much of the information contained in patient histories comes from patients themselves. Think of the various consultations patients may have before being diagnosed, interviews in which they provide medical information of vital importance to the physician; or questionnaires patients answer in population studies, or forms patients have to complete in order to apply for services. All of these are examples of how medical knowledge and communication also flows bottom-up.

Specialized *and* popular

The transmission of medical knowledge takes place in a wide range of situations from highly specialized research papers communicating the results of a study to newspaper articles giving an account of or commenting on a given discovery, invention, or controversy in the medical and health sectors. Between the research article and the newspaper article there is a wide spectrum of communicative situations of decreasing degrees of specialization.

Formal *and* informal

Formal communication in the medical field might involve published papers or presentations at conferences. But like any other social activity, medicine involves a wide variety of communicative practices many of which take place in informal situations: researchers talk to each other in order to share information of all kinds, plan experiments, comment on results, and so on. Likewise physicians in hospitals also talk to each other about patients, or write informal notes to remember things. Patients also express themselves informally when they consult their consultants or when they talk to other patients who suffer from the same illness.

These are just a few examples of the many informal situations in which medical communication takes place.

Oral *and* written

Medical knowledge can be generated and communicated not only in written form but also orally. When a patient and a physician exchange information in the consulting room, or when researchers swap ideas in the laboratory or the clinic or during a coffee break at a conference, they are all producing and communicating medical knowledge orally. That knowledge will probably be stored and further elaborated in written form. In the first case, the patient's comments may be written down and stored in her/his clinical history. In the second case, many of the oral interchanges between the investigators of a research team will be developed further in the form of a laboratory report, which in its turn may give rise to a conference presentation and, if the research is relevant enough, to an article published in a specialized journal.

This book is mainly concerned with formal written communication not restricted to experts, but including all possible participants and communicative purposes.

Our vision of medical knowledge and communication assumes that they are social activities, and therefore influence and are influenced by the broader social and cultural context in which they occur. Compare, for instance, the following texts on anorexia nervosa published with different readerships in mind:

Academic

Source: Russell, Gerald F. (1982) 'Anorexia Nervosa', in Wyngaarden, James B. and Lloyd H. Smith (eds) *Cecil Textbook of Medicine* (16th ed) (2), Philadelphia, London, Toronto, Mexico City, Rio de Janeiro, Sydney, Tokyo: Igaku-Shoin and Saunders International Edition. 1379.

DEFINITION. Anorexia nervosa is a prolonged illness principally affecting young girls after puberty. It is characterized by severe weight loss which is self-induced, amenorrhea, and a specific psychopatholgy (…)
ETIOLOGY
    The cause of anorexia nervosa is unknown. Little is known about genetic aspects: morbidity is higher amongst sisters of patients (6.6 per cent), and concordance for the illness has been described in identical twins, but these observations are also explicable by the similarity of the home environment (…) the prevalence may be high in groups at special risk: 1 of 250 among schoolgirls aged16 or over in England (Crisp et al) (…)

Professional

Source: Castro, J., A. Gila, J. Puig, S. Rodriguez and J. Toro (2004) 'Predictors of rehospitalization after total weight recovery in adolescents with anorexia nervosa', International *Journal Eating Disorders*, July, 36(1): 22-30.

Predictors of rehospitalization after total weight recovery in adolescents with anorexia nervosa.

OBJECTIVE: The current study analyzed the variables related to rehospitalization after total weight recovery in adolescents with anorexia nervosa. METHOD: One hundred and one patients first admitted for inpatient treatment, aged 11-19 years, were followed up for 12 months after discharge. RESULTS: Twenty-five subjects (24.8%) required readmission after complete weight recovery and 76 (75.2%) did not. Duration of disorder, weight loss, body mass index at first admission, and global body image distortion were similar in the two groups (…)

Mainstream

Source: ANAD (National Association of Anorexia Nervosa and Associated Disorders) http://www.anad.org/site/anadweb/

Welcome to the National Association of Anorexia Nervosa and Associated Disorders – ANAD.

General Information

FACTS ABOUT EATING DISORDERS:

EATING DISORDERS ARE WIDESPREAD AND DESTRUCTIVE

- Eating disorders cause immeasurable suffering for victims and families.
- Eating disorders have reached epidemic levels in America: all segments of society, young and old, rich and poor, all minorities, including African American and Latino
- Seven million women
- One million men
  (...)

Popular

Source: Larsen, Joanne MS RD LD (1995-2003) *Ask the Dietitian* SM Copyright ©, http://www.dietitian.com/anorexia.html

I'm so glad I found your site on the Internet! Eating disorders are hardly acknowledged in the Far East and I'm starting to get really worried about my best friend.

My friend has been on this crazy diet for six months since we started freshman year at law school and she's lost 17 kilos (37.4 lbs.)! She used to be a nicely rounded at 60 kg (132 lbs.) and 166 cm (5 ft 5) but now she weighs 43.5 kilos (96 lbs.). Is this too thin?

Her work has always been excellent and she was always popular, but now she's really changed. Sure she has a boyfriend and has even been offered a modeling job, but I got real scared (..)

Traditionally, medical language has been regarded in the same way as any other kind of scientific language: objective, neutral and non-rhetorical, whose only function was to transmit information, a so-called 'referential' function. In this traditional, received image of medical language, words and texts are detached from society and from the individual. As a consequence, they contain no cultural or ideological references, and have a uniform and impersonal style. Furthermore, each concept is represented by one – and only one – term, (in the jargon of linguists 'univocal') and concepts are precise and remain stable and unchanging over time.

Received view	**Critical view**
Referential function	Any function
Objective	Intersubjective
Neutral	Focalized, metaphorical
Non-rhetorical	Rhetorical
Absence of cultural and ideological elements	Cultural and ideological elements
Uniform and impersonal style	Variety of styles
Univocal terminology	Polysemy and synonymy
Conceptual precision and stability	Conceptual variation

Figure 2.1. Received and critical views of medical language

Medical texts may include characteristics of different text types, degrees of formality and both a subjective and objective orientation – compare, for instance, the *abstract* and the *discussion* in an original article, or the mixture of academic language and non-specialized explanations in this pharmaceutical leaflet:

> Like many medicines, Bendrofluazide tablets may occasionally cause side-effects in some patients... These may include ... feeling faint when getting up (postural hypotension) ... inability to maintain an erection (this effect is reversible)... pancreatitis (inflammation of the pancreas causing severe abdominal pain)...

That so-called scientific objectivity may be a controversial issue comes across clearly in the choice of words or expressions motivated by political correction or in the search for positive connotations in the following guidelines for authors (*Neurology*, January 1995), similar to those for most publications:

- It is easy to mix fact and opinion: keep the Results and Discussion separate.
- Don't overuse italics for emphasis. A page peppered with different type styles confuses the eye and interrupts smooth reading.
- The routine mention of a patient's skin color or ethnic origin is usually superfluous and should appear in a case report only if later addressed in the discussion or if potentially useful for future studies, as with skin color in a hypertensive population.
- Do not use the phrase "in man"; "human" is the appropriate alternative.
- We are accused of dehumanizing patients. Consider the following:

instead of	use
case	patient
male or female	man or woman
male or female children	boys or girls
pediatric population	children

Our approach to medical knowledge and communication as social activity implies a critical vision of the language. Participants use language to achieve their communicative goals, which are not limited to just transmitting factual information. So medical language can – and indeed does – carry out a variety of functions (see the genres presented in this chapter). For those who are familiar with the jargon, it is the result of interpersonal interaction (intersubjective) in which individuals communicate with each other from a specific point of view (focalized) by means of metaphors (see 3.3 and 5.4) and a rich variety of rhetorical and stylistic resources. In addition medical language contains cultural and ideological elements. This is especially visible in the language used to communicate with patients. As far as terminology is concerned, polysemy, synonymy (see chapter 7) and conceptual variation are at least as common as univocal, precise and stable terms. How does all this affect medical translators and the way they work? Well, first and foremost, it should indicate that translators bear in mind who is likely to read their translations and why. The next section explores this aspect.

2.2 Participants in medical communication and their communicative purposes

Before starting to draft our target text (see chapter 4), it is important to consider who is likely to read it and in which circumstances, so we should give some thought to the following points:

- Educational and professional background – in general it is easier to write for readers whose educational and professional background is sound
- Levels of knowledge and experience – the reader's previous knowledge about a particular topic determines the degree of explicitness and amount of explanation required when writing the target text
- Purposes and applications of the information – readers read texts in order to able to do things or find out about them
- Linguistic abilities – for a variety of reasons, some readers may not have a good command of their own language when used in non-colloquial, unfamiliar contexts
- Familiarity with specialized terminology – when shared by the reader, terminology is highly convenient because it saves time and effort in the writing process; when not shared, however, the use of specialized terminology can be a communicative barrier for the reader
- Reading context – the physical and psychological conditions in which the readers read the text
- Broader cultural context – the country where they live; the particular values and beliefs about health held in that country; the organization of the health system, the University system, the research system, and so forth.

As we have already seen, many different people are involved in medical communication. For practical and pedagogical purposes, attention may be focused on five reader profiles: general readers, patients, students, health professionals and researchers. These five profiles correspond to different degrees of specialization and, therefore, of complexity for the translator. Although they all read for practical reasons (all are functional readers), each of them wants the information for different reasons and uses it in different ways:

Reader profile	*Application of information*
General reader	Preventing disease
Patient	Treating disease
Student	Becoming a health professional
Health professional	Implementing knowledge
Researcher	Advancing knowledge

Figure 2.2. Reader profile and application of information

Now it would be helpful to consider the way readers read functional texts. According to Wright (1999: 96), three stages can be distinguished: access to information, interpretation and application.

Access
- reader asks questions
- reader skip-searches for information likely to contain the answer(s)

Interpretation
- reader understands the verbal information
- reader understands the graphic information
- reader integrates verbal and graphic information
- reader infers personal relevance
- reader infers author's agenda

Application
- reader integrates understanding with personal beliefs and attitudes
- reader determines appropriate decisions and actions
- reader devises an action plan – i.e. subgoals and necessary steps
- reader carries out all steps in plan, monitoring outcomes
- if monitoring yields a mismatch between subgoals and attainment, reader formulates a new question and recycles from Access

Figure 2.3. Summary of how people read functional texts
(Wright, 1999: 96)

In accordance with the reader's profile, needs and application, medical authors choose a particular genre (see 2.4 Articulating written communication through genres) to convey their message. For example, if the reader is a scientist doing research in the treatment of a particular disease, authors may choose the research article to communicate their own research. If the reader is a patient, authors will have to choose a different genre (probably the summary for patients) to communicate the same message.

When translating research articles to be published in specialized journals, medical translators should note that two specific reading processes may take place:

- *refereeing* in which independent anonymous referees select the articles that will be published in the journal on the basis of relevance of content and good style.
- *reviewing* in which experts in the subject matter of the article summarize and evaluate its findings.

Task 1. Analyzing your readership

1) Read the text below and analyze its likely readership by exploring the following questions:

- Who are the readers?
- Do you think they belong to a profession or social group? Why will they read the text?
- How much do you think they know about the topic of the text?
- In which context will they read the text and for which purposes?
- What should they know, think or be able to do after reading the text?

Hyperlipoproteinemia (hyperlipidemia) is abnormally high levels of lipids (cholesterol, triglycerides, or both) carried by lipoproteins in the blood.

Levels of lipoproteins (and therefore lipids, particularly LDL cholesterol) increase slightly as people age. Levels are normally slightly higher in men than in women, but levels increase in women after menopause. The increase in levels of lipoproteins that occurs with age can result in hyperlipoproteinemia and increase the risk of atherosclerosis. (A high level of HDL — the good — cholesterol is beneficial and is not considered a disorder.) [...]

Treatment

Usually, the best treatment for people who have high cholesterol or triglyceride levels is to lose weight if they are overweight, stop smoking if they smoke, decrease the total amount of fat and cholesterol in their diet, increase physical activity, and, if necessary, take a lipid-lowering drug.

A diet low in fats and cholesterol can lower the LDL cholesterol level. Experts recommend limiting calories from fat to no more than 25 to 35% of the total calories consumed over several days.

The type of fat consumed is also important. Fats may be saturated, polyunsaturated, or monounsaturated. Saturated fats increase cholesterol levels more than other forms of fat. Saturated fats should provide no more than 7 to 10% of total calories consumed each day. Polyunsaturated fats (which include omega-3 fats and omega-6 fats) and monounsaturated fats may help decrease levels of triglycerides and LDL cholesterol in the blood. The fat content of most foods is included on the label of the container.

2) Go to <http://www.merck.com/mmhe/sec12/ch157/ch157b.html> [...] and try to find out more about these issues.

2.3 Relationships among texts in written communication

Written texts in any communicative situation can be interrelated in three basic ways: referential, functional, and generic. As will be seen in the rest of the book, these relationships are often of relevance to the medical translator.

Referential intertextuality

Directly or indirectly, medical texts — and indeed all texts — contain references and information from other texts. For example, a textbook on a university course contains information that comes from well-established sources of medical knowledge such as treatises, encyclopaedias, as well as from research papers and revision articles that contribute to updating medical knowledge. This is called referential intertextuality and it can best be seen in direct citations and bibliographic references.

Functional intertextuality

Different texts dealing with the same topic may have different functions. In the example above, a University textbook may contain information from a given set of research articles but it is used for a different purpose: to support the teaching-learning process of future health professionals. Other genres fulfill other functions: an editorial on smoking and heart diseases in a research journal critically comments on one or several original articles on that subject; a leading original article on breast cancer and a specific drug may give rise to a summary for patients or a newspaper article on that same topic, but with different functions.

We will call this textual relationship between texts functional intertextuality. Functional intertextuality underlines the fact that genres are dependent on each other as far as communication is concerned because each of them covers specific needs of writers and readers, as can be seen in the flow diagram below:

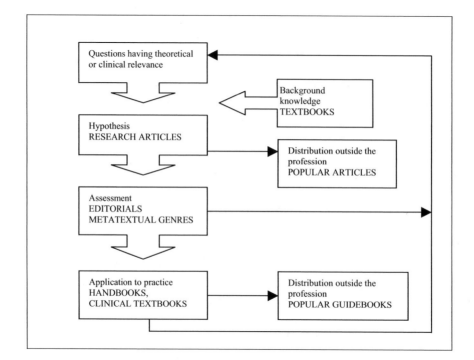

Figure 2.4. Functional hierarchy of medical genres
(Vihla, 1999: 128)

Generic intertextuality

Different texts dealing with different topics may carry out exactly the same function and share the same formal features. For instance, an editorial in any medical journal – regardless of the topic it deals with – comments on the research contained in other articles, tries to provoke critical discussion and, typically, has no fixed section and subsection headings. Likewise, any patient information leaflet

− regardless of the particular medicinal product − is used to guide the patient as how to take the medicine (see 'Patient Information Leaflet' below). This type of relationship among texts that share the same function and the same formal characteristics is called generic intertextuality.

2.4 Articulating written communication through genres

What is a genre?

As has been pointed out, texts share participants, functions, and the situations in which they are used as well as formal conventions with many other similar texts; that is, any text belongs to a more or less recognizable textual genre (i.e. editorial, original article, review article, case report, book review, text book, clinical guide, etc.). Following Bazerman (1998: 24), we could define genre as:

> [...] not just [...] the formal characteristics that one must observe so as to be recognised as correctly following the visible rules and expectations. Genre more fundamentally is a kind of activity to be carried out in a recognisable textual space. That activity embodies relations with the readers and kinds of messages to be developed in order to carry out generically appropriate intentions and interactions − to complete the rhetorical and social possibilities of the genre. Thus genre presents an opportunity space for realising certain kinds of activities, meanings, and relations. Genre exists only in the recognition and deployment of typicality by writers and readers − it is the recognisable shape by which participation is enacted and understood.

According to this definition, an original article as a genre is not just a set of formal characteristics − structure, length, tenor, degree of specialization of the information contained, and so on − that must be fulfilled, but is also a communicative activity carried out by researchers whose purpose is to convince readers of their conclusions, gain prestige, make the discipline advance, and so on.

Thus, written communication in health practices covers more than just the purely expository research genres. According to the overall rhetorical purpose of the writer, we can distinguish three basic types of genres.

Overall rhetorical purpose of the writer	Examples of genres
Instructional: give instructions to readers so that they carry out certain actions	Clinical guidelines, patient information leaflet, manual.
Expository: provide information to readers	Anatomical atlas, treatise, review article, case report, first part of an informed consent.
Argumentative: convince readers	Medical editorial, original article, poster in health campaign.

Figure 2.5. Examples of genres according to the main rhetorical purpose of the writer

In addition, we can distinguish further medical genres according to their overall social function:

Overall social function	Examples of genres
Preventing disease, educating the general public, creating awareness of risks, etc...	Genres in institutional campaigns such as press releases, information for patients, etc...
Carrying out domestic actions such as following a diet, or a treatment...	Diet, patient information leaflet, etc...
Communicating new discoveries to non-specialized readerships	Newspaper article, summary for patient, mainstream book, non specialist manual, etc...
Teaching and learning how to become a health professional	Text-book, manual, encyclopaedia, anatomical atlas, etc...
Carrying out clinical practice, implementing new techniques in clinical practice	Patient's history, guide of practice, manual, etc...
Selling products to professionals	Advertisement, leaflets and other promotional material
Communicating new research to specialized audiences	Original article, review article, scientific editorial, etc...

Figure 2.6. Genres according to overall social function

Bridging communication gaps within the same language

Some genres are used to store information and transmit it among members of the same knowledge community, be it professional – researchers, physicians, and so on – or non-professional – patients, general public. For example, a research article is conceived of as a genre for storing highly specialized information so that it is available in the future and for transmitting it to the community of researchers in that particular field of research. Likewise, the clinical history of a patient is a macrogenre used to facilitate clinical exchange between and activity in health professionals during treatment.

Some other genres are used to bridge communication gaps between speakers of the same language that belong to different knowledge communities.

Communication gaps	*Some genres used to bridge them*
Between patients and physicians (patients need to understand clearly the details of their disease: mechanism, causes, risks, treatment, etc...)	Fact sheet for patients; patient information leaflet.
Between patients and researchers (patients need to and have the right to know the progress of research in the disease that affects them...)	Summary of research articles for patients; popularizing article; press release.
Between physicians and researchers (physicians need to apply advances in research in order to improve clinical practice and patients' treatment...)	Clinical guidelines; review article.

Figure 2.7. Bridging communication gaps through genres

Why should we pay attention to genres and not just to texts when translating?

In professional practice, a translation is required and commissioned when there is a communicative niche – in our case, the need of a text – within a target communicative situation, and more specifically, within a target genre. Thus, when translating, target genre knowledge and skills are key elements, from both a communicative and a formal point of view (García and Montalt, 2002). As medical translators, we are especially interested in genres because our translation strategies, procedures and decisions may depend on four factors:

a) *Comprehension.* Understanding the source text depends on the profile and previous knowledge of the reader to whom the genre is typically addressed. A medical translation student will be cognitively and communicatively closer to some genres – such as a patient information leaflet – than to others – such as a clinical trial protocol. Socializing with genres with which we are not familiar is vital for the adequate comprehension of specialized texts.

b) *Translation process.* Knowing about structural elements in different genres enables us to anticipate the type of information we should be looking for as we read the source text and draft the target text (see chapter 4).

c) *Interlinguistic differences.* Even if the target text belongs to the same genre as the source text, there might be important differences in the way it is realized in the target culture.

d) *Genre shifts.* Depending on the translation assignment, the target text may or may not belong to the same genre as the source text (see 4.6 Genre shifts: Drafting heterofunctional translations).

Task 2. Spotting genres

Read the following excerpt:

Without humor, life would undeniably be less exhilarating. Indeed, the ability to comprehend and find a joke funny plays a defining role in the human condition, essentially helping us to communicate ideas, attract partners, boost mood, and even cope in times of trauma and stress.

Can you guess where it was originally written?:

(a) A newspaper article?
(b) A specialized medical text?
(c) A resource book for comedians?

The answer is (b), although it could probably have been the first paragraph of any of the above. They are the introductory words to the article "Humour modulates the mesolimbic reward centers" (Mobbs, D. *et al.*, in *Neuron*, 2003).

Now compare the text (above) with the title and the first two paragraphs of the same text (below) as it was rewritten by Helen Pearson for *Nature* (4 December 2003):

> **Jokes activate same brain region as cocaine**
> *Humour tickles drug centre that gives hedonistic high*
>
> There's truth in the maxim 'laughter is a drug'. A comic cartoon fired up the same brain centre as a shot of cocaine, researchers are reporting.
> A team at Stanford University in California asked lab mates, spouses and friends to select the wittiest newspaper cartoons from a portfolio. They showed the winning array to 16 volunteers while peering inside their heads by functional magnetic resonance imaging (fMRI).
> The cartoons activated the same reward circuits in the brain that are tickled by cocaine, money or a pretty face, the neuroscientists found. One brain region in particular, the nucleus accumbens, lit up seconds after a rib-tickler but remained listless after a lacklustre cartoon.
>
> Let us now return to the specialized medical text. Continue reading it (below) to spot the differences in register, conventions of presentation, vocabulary and phraseology between this text and the one written for *Nature* (above) inspired by Mobbs et al:
>
> … (Dixon, 1980; Gavrilovic et al., 2003; Martin, Neuhoff and Schaefer, 2002; Nezlek and Derks, 2001). These beneficial manifestations are complemented at the physiological level where humor (i.e., the perception that something is funny; McGhee, 1971) is thought to have numerous salutary effects, including acting as a natural stress antagonist and possibly enhancing the cardiovascular, immune, and endocrine systems (Bennett et al., 2003; Berk et al., 1989; Fredrickson and Levenson, 1998; Fry, 1992; Lefcourt et al., 1990). It is therefore apparent that developing a sophisticated understanding of the discrete neural systems that modulate humor appreciation is of both social and clinical relevance.
>
> As a last step, translate the two different texts as if they were assignments from two journals with different readerships in your country. If your country is English-speaking, you may carry out an intralingual translation (English to English).

2.5 Some common medical genres

As we have seen, written medical communication in formal contexts is carried out through well-established genres. Researching medical genres and getting to know them well – their communicative purpose; the situations where they are used; their participants' motivations and expectations; and their typical structure and form – is a key to successful medical translation. In this section we look at some medical genres as examples of what the medical translator normally has to deal with in professional practice. In particular we look at the following: fact sheet for patients, informed consent, patient information leaflet, summary of product characteristics, clinical guide, case report, review article, standard operating procedures, clinical trial protocol, and advertisement.

Fact Sheet for Patients (FSP)

Patient education is a critical factor not only in controlling – and hopefully over-coming – a particular disease or condition, but also in preventing it. Traditionally the only source of information for patients has been the doctor in the context of the consulting room. This is no longer the case. In the era of the Internet and of the democratization of medical knowledge, patients have access to quality information about their diseases. Being well informed enables them to contribute to their own health and well-being.

A FSP – also referred to as 'patient leaflet', 'patient information brochure', and 'patient brochure' – is normally issued by a health organization: a local, national or international governmental body; a patients' association; a professional association; a research institute; a hospital; a medical society. It is intended to provide patients with the main – and most relevant – information about a particular disease or condition – symptoms, causes, treatment, and so forth – medicine, or diagnostic procedure.

FSPs are normally written by health professionals in such a way that patients and their relatives can understand the content of the text. The information they contain often comes from highly reliable, well-established medical information sources such as clinical handbooks, treatises, revision articles, and medical textbooks. In other words, FSPs are re-elaborations and re-contextualizations of previous texts belonging to more specialized genres. See 'Figure 2.4 Functional hierarchy of medical genres (Vihla, 1999: 128)' above, in which FSPs would fall in the communication space of 'Distribution outside the profession'.

FSPs present information in an-easy-to-read, concise way. Hence the headings of the different sections express succinctly the most relevant aspects of the disease. These are organized hierarchically, starting from the most basic ones such as defining the disease and its causes to presenting the most recent research being done and outlining some of the findings published in international research journals. To become familiar with the typical sections of most FSPs, go to section 3 of chapter 4 (4.3 Composing your target text).

As far as terminology is concerned, in FSPs medical terms are accompanied by explanations, as in the following examples:

- Some experts contend that the best approach is to immediately perform specific diagnostic testing, such as an upper *endoscopy* (a test in which a patient swallows a thin flexible tube with a camera that shows pictures of the stomach).

- The disease flares up from time to time and becomes active (*relapse*).
- The *ureters* are tubes that carry urine from the kidney to the bladder.

See examples of this genre

In the following links you will find examples of texts belonging to this genre. Read some of them so as to become familiar with their communicative purpose, structure, types of information contained in each part of the structure, phraseology, terminology, style, and tenor.

- <http://www.who.int/mediacentre/factsheets/en>
- <http://patients.uptodate.com>
- <http://www.patients.co.uk>
- <http://familydoctor.org>
- <http://medlineplus.gov>

A note on tasks 3 to 9:

To have a broader, more useful understanding of this genre, find examples of it in your target language. Do the same for all the genres in this section. Collect examples so that you can use them as parallel texts in the future.

Task 3. Transforming a manual for physicians into a fact sheet for patients

1) Go to <http://www.merck.com/mrkshared/mmanual/section4/chapter42/42b.jsp> and read the text about acute viral hepatitis carefully. You will probably have to do some research on concepts and terms you are not familiar with.
2) Decide which information you would select for a fact sheet for patients of this text.
3) Decide how you are going to present specialized terms so that your reader will understand them. For help on this front, go to chapter 7 and read section '7.5 De-terminologizing the text.'
4) Go to chapter 4 and read section 4.6 Genre shifts: Drafting heterofunctional translations.
5) Write a FSP in your target language using the methodology suggested in chapter 4. Choose the structure that best suits the communicative needs of your target reader. For this purpose you can use the information provided in 'Figure 4.6 Comparison of two structures of fact sheets for patients' in chapter 4.

Informed Consent (IC)

The informed consent fulfils two main purposes. On the one hand, it can be used to express the patient's written consent to a surgical or medical procedure or other course of treatment, given after the physician has explained the potential benefits and risks, and discussed any possible alternative treatment. The concept of informed consent is based on the principle that a physician has a duty to disclose to patients information that allows them to make a reasonable decision regarding their own treatment. On the other hand, an informed consent is also required for participation in clinical studies.

Experimentation on human beings is a key aspect for the progress of medical research. New drugs, procedures and techniques can only be fully validated if they have been tested on people. In the course of recent history, however, experimentation on humans has been immorally abused. The judgment by the war crimes tribunal at Nuremberg laid down 10 principles known as the Nuremberg Code (1947) to which physicians must conform when carrying out experiments on human subjects. The first principle of this code states the following:

> The voluntary consent of the human subject is absolutely essential. This means that the person involved should have legal capacity to give consent; should be so situated as to be able to exercise free power of choice, without the intervention of any element of force, fraud, deceit, duress, overreaching, or other ulterior form of constraint or coercion; and should have sufficient knowledge and comprehension of the elements of the subject matter involved as to enable him to make an understanding and enlightened decision. This latter element requires that before the acceptance of an affirmative decision by the experimental subject there should be made known to him the nature, duration, and purpose of the experiment; the method and means by which it is to be conducted; all inconveniences and hazards reasonably to be expected; and the effects upon his health or person which may possibly come from his participation in the experiment. The duty and responsibility for ascertaining the quality of the consent rests upon each individual who initiates, directs, or engages in the experiment. It is a personal duty and responsibility which may not be delegated to another with impunity.
> (Source: http://bmj.bmjjournals.com/cgi/content full/313/7070/ 1448? ijkey=d090fb639d942fd6accb9726 29ac8d5a71a96d78&keytype2=tf_ ipsecsha)

Likewise, one of the basic principles of the Declaration of Helsinki adopted by the 18th World Medical Association General Assembly (Helsinki, Finland, June 1964) states:

In any research on human beings, each potential subject must be adequately informed of the aims, methods, sources of funding, any possible conflicts of interest, institutional affiliations of the researcher, the anticipated benefits and potential risks of the study and the discomfort it may entail. The subject should be informed of the right to abstain from participation in the study or to withdraw consent to participate at any time without reprisal. After ensuring that the subject has understood the information, the physician should then obtain the subject's freely-given informed consent, preferably in writing. If the consent cannot be obtained in writing, the non-written consent must be formally documented and witnessed.

These two legal texts clearly state the main purpose of the informed consent: that a person – when asked to participate in a clinical study – can exercise free power of choice based on knowledge and comprehension of the elements of the subject matter involved.

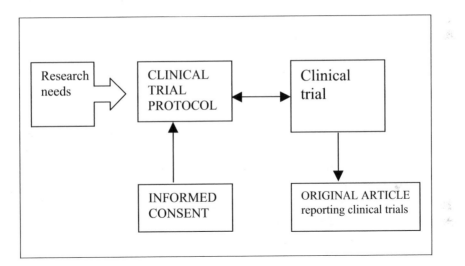

Figure 2.8. Systems of genres: research that involves human experimentation

A consent form written in a language too technical or containing jargon will often be deemed incomprehensible and intimidating for a potential participant. We must make every effort to write for the intended audience by using language appropriate for the participants' age group and educational background, and use lay language when possible.

With regard to structure and types of information, an informed consent has two main parts. The first part is informative and contains details about the study to be carried out. The second part consists of the consent itself, that is, the authorization.

Although different organizations adapt the format of the IC to their particular needs, the informative part of most IC contains the following data:

- The background, nature, justification, and purpose of the study
- The institutional affiliations of the researchers
- The institutions that promote the study, and also the institutions that support or approve the study
- The method and means by which the study is to be conducted, mainly the type of clinical study, the drug or device to be used, the duration of the study, and the number and location of the participants
- The specific participation required of the patient in the study, such as interviews and tests the patient has to go through, as well as the number of doses and strength of the drug in the case of pharmacological trials
- The discomforts and risks to be expected from the study
- The benefits to be expected from the study
- The availability of medical treatment should complications occur
- The opportunity to withdraw at any time without affecting any future care at the participating institution
- Information about insurance
- Information about confidentiality.

Figure 2.9. Types of information in the first part of informed consents

As far as the second part is concerned, the key element is the authorization, that is, the signature of the person giving consent, which is typically written in the first person singular. In the signature section there is usually a clear statement that the document is signed on condition that the subject may withdraw at any time. It is also stated that the person signing has read carefully and understood all the particulars of the study, has received enough information, has been able to ask questions about it, and has had the opportunity to talk to a researcher involved in the study. A witness to the signature of the document is normally required. When the participants in the study are children, their parents' signatures are required. Opinions differ about whether children and the mentally ill, for example, can really be considered capable of giving truly informed consent.

Title of the study: _____

Code of the study: _____

I have carefully read the information contained above, and I understand fully my rights as a potential subject in this study. The researcher has explained the study to me and answered my questions. I know what will be asked of me. I understand the purpose of this study. If I do not participate, there will be no penalty or loss of rights. I can stop participating at any time, even after I have started.

I agree to participate in this study.

Date: _____

Signature: _____ Name _____
    (patient)

Signature: _____ Name _____
    (researcher)

Signature: _____ Name _____
    (witness)

Figure 2.10. A simplified version of the authorization section of an informed consent

See examples of this genre

In the following links you will find examples of texts belonging to this genre. Read some of them so as to become familiar with their communicative purpose, structure, types of information contained in each part of the structure, phraseology, terminology, style, and tenor.

- <http://www.who.int/rpc/research_ethics/informed_consent/en>
- <http://www.niams.nih.gov/rtac/clinical/observ.htm>
- <http://www.nihtraining.com/ohsrsite/info/sheet6.html>
- <http://www.ccsu.edu/humanstudies/Sample%20Consent%20Form.htm>
- <http://talkbank.org/share/consent.html>

Task 4. Exploring informed consents

Using the advanced search facilities of Google or any other search engine, find informed consents in your target language and answer the following questions:

- Are they used for giving consent to participate in clinical trials or to accept a given procedure or treatment in clinical practice?
- What types of information can you find in them? Check them against the list in Figure 2.9 above.
- What linguistic formulae are used in the consent sections? Who signs them?

Patient Information Leaflet (PIL)

If you have ever been prescribed a medicine or bought an over-the-counter medicine, you will probably be familiar with this genre. The patient information leaflet – also called 'information leaflet', 'package insert', 'patient package insert', 'consumer medicine information' – is the document enclosed in the outer sales package of a medicinal product and is written in the national language(s) of the country where it is sold. The PIL is one of the most common genres in medical communication and translation.

PILs are issued by pharmaceutical companies in accordance with the requirements of the drug regulatory agencies in each country and, in the case of European Community countries, also in accordance with the European Medicinal Agency (EMEA). In the United States, the regulatory agency is the FDA (Food and Drug Administration).

PILs are summarized and simplified versions of longer, more complex documents addressed to experts that are produced for the development and approval of medicines, such as core data sheets and summary of product characteristics (SPC) (see figure 2.9 below). As far as the European context is concerned, in the 'Guidelines on Summary of Product Characteristics' (1999) the European Commission states: 'The content of the package leaflet must be consistent with the SPC but in a wording that can be easily understood by non-professionals.'

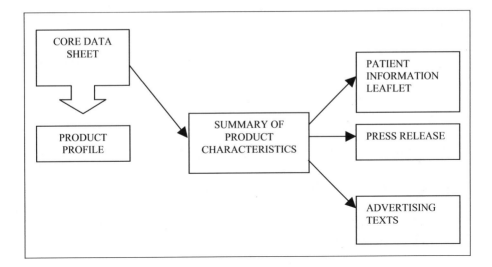

*Figure 2.11. Systems of genres: main genres in
the pharmaceutical context*

In the case of the European Union, drug dossiers published by the European Medicinal Agency contain summaries of product characteristics addressed to prescribers as well as the packaging information relevant to the patients. Packaging information is made up of PILs and labelling information. Labelling information is the text printed on both the outer package – containers, usually cardboard boxes – and the direct packaging, e.g. blister packs, ampoules, bottles, tubes, sachets, of a medicine. Labelling information is also subject to national regulatory requirements.

After the doctor has prescribed the medicine, the patient alone is responsible for taking it as directed; that is, in a safe and effective way. Safety and efficacy depend not only on the indications and contraindications of the medicine – it is the doctor's decision which medicine a particular patient needs – but also on taking it exactly as prescribed. Taking more or less medicine than prescribed or taking it under certain circumstances may be a cause for concern. Hence the importance of accuracy and clarity when translating PILs, especially the section devoted to posology and method of administration.

Dose

Use a 5 ml plastic spoon or oral syringe available from the pharmacist to take the syrup. The usual doses are:
Children 2 to 6 years: 2.5 ml (1 mg) to 5 ml (2 mg) three or four times daily.
Children 6 to 12 years: 5 ml (2 mg) three or four times daily.
Children over 12 years: 5 ml (2 mg) to 10 ml (4 mg) three or four times daily.
Adults: 5 ml (2 mg) to 20 ml (8 mg) up to four times daily.

*IT IS VERY IMPORTANT that you keep to your doctor's instructions as to how much syrup to take and how often to take it. DO NOT TAKE more than you were told to.
*Keep taking your medicine for as long as your doctor tells you. Do not stop just because you feel better.
*You may find it helps to wipe the neck of the bottle after use.

Figure 2.12. Example of the posology section of a PIL

PILs not only remind patients of the dosage and method of administration, but also give them the following information:

- *The name of the product*. At the beginning of the leaflet, the trade name of the medicinal product is stated together with the strength and the pharmaceutical form. This is normally followed by the generic name of the active substance
- *The pharmaceutical form*. The form in which the medicine is prepared for human use: tablets, syrup, aerosol, capsules, and so forth
- *The marketing authorization holder*. In the target text, this information may have to be replaced with the data of the target marketplace national brand in the case of multinational companies
- *The composition of the medicinal product*. The qualitative and quantitative composition of the active substance and the full qualitative composition of the excipients
- *The pharmacotherapeutic classification*. According to the WHO's ATC/DDD system. See <http://www.whocc.no/atcddd>
- *Characteristics*. A description of the properties of the medicine, as in this example: 'ACE inhibitors reduce constriction of blood vessels, which makes it easier for the blood to flow through them.'
- *Indications*. The use of the medicine, as in this example: 'Acepril is used to

lower high blood pressure or to help the heart pump blood around the body and in the treatment of heart failure. It is also used to treat people after a heart attack [...]'

- *Contraindications*. This section states who should not take the medicine. It might be children, the elderly, pregnant and nursing mothers, and special patient populations such as patients with kidney or liver impairment

- *Undesirable effects*. They are normally listed in decreasing order of seriousness. Irrespective of their frequency, very serious, typical, undesirable effects of the product are often mentioned first or are specially emphasized, as in 'Very occasionally these effects may be severe causing swelling, shock and collapse. You should seek medical advice IMMEDIATELY if you experience these effects'. Undesirable effects are usually subdivided according to seriousness and frequency, or according to symptom type. To avoid creating excessive anxiety in patients, special attention should be paid to the way language is modulated through hedging expressions such as the ones italicized in this sentence 'This medicine *sometimes* causes unwanted effects in *some* people. These effects *may* include [...]'

- *Interactions*. Effects of other products – not only other medicines but also food and alcohol if relevant – on the particular medicine are described in this section

- *Special warnings and precautions*. This section may contain information about the influence of the drug on the patient's behaviour, masked symptoms, intolerance of specific materials, and many more

- *Package sizes*. All package sizes approved are given here

- *Storing*. The maximum in-use shelf life is stated together with the storage conditions

- *Date of last revision*.

In PILs technical terms are often accompanied by explanations or even simply avoided in order to enable patients to understand unfamiliar concepts better, as in the following example: 'Non-steroideal anti-inflammatory agents (a type of painkiller, e.g. indometacin, aspirin)'

Owing to marketing strategies, multinational companies sometimes sell their products with different trade names in different countries. Therefore, we should check whether the medicine is commercialized with the same trade name in the target marketplace. Just to give a few examples, the pharmaceutical company GlaxoSmithKline commercializes the medicine containing sumatriptan as the active ingredient with the trade name 'Imitrex' in the United States, and 'Imigran' in the United Kingdom, Spain, Italy, and other countries. Likewise, the paroxetine sold by this pharmaceutical company is commercialized as 'Paxil' in the US and 'Seroxat' in the UK and other European countries. Roche's bromazepam is called 'Lexatín' in Spain, 'Lexotan' in the United States, the United Kingdom, Portugal, and Brazil, 'Lexomil' in France, 'Lectopam' in Canada, 'Lexotanil' in Germany, and 'Lexotán' in Mexico. (See chapter 7 on synonymy).

It is also important for medical translators to bear in mind that some countries prefer using national nomenclatures instead of the international one recommended by the World Health Organization, International Nonpropietary Names, INN. Therefore, the generic name used may vary from one country to another when naming active ingredients of the medicine in the name of the product section of the PIL.

In order to comply with regulations on the accessibility of PILs brought in recently in some countries, pharmaceutical companies are starting to offer PILs in Braille and other formats, such as large print and CD-Rom, that enable visually impaired people to access information about their treatment.

See examples of this genre

In the following links you will find examples of texts belonging to this genre. Read some of them so as to become familiar with their communicative purpose, structure, types of information contained in each part of the structure, phraseology, terminology, style, and tenor.

- <http://www.emea.eu.int> (in 20 European languages)
- <http://emc.medicines.org.uk>
- <www.gsk.com>
- <http://www.roche.com/home.html>

Task 5. Comparing PILs in different languages and from different companies

1) Choose a medicine you have used recently or simply one you are familiar with. Read the PIL in your target language.
2) Find the PILs for the same medicine in the other language or languages you use as a translator.
3) Compare the texts. Are there any differences as far as structure, headings, style, tenor and terminology are concerned? Try to explain the differences.
4) Now look for PILs in your target language for four medicines commercialized by four different pharmaceutical companies.
5) Compare them asking the following questions: Are there any differences as far as symbols, visual elements, structure, headings, style, tenor and terminology are concerned? Which of them is the clearest and most readable? Why?

Summary of Product Characteristics (SPC)

In order to commercialize any medicine in the European Union, a marketing authorization must be issued by the European Medicines Agency (http://www.emea.eu.int). One of the documents attached to every application for marketing authorization is the proposal for a summary of product characteristics. The SPC together with the package leaflet, constitutes Part I B of the dossier which is required by the authorities. This document summarizes the main characteristics of a medicinal product from different points of view: pharmacological, chemical, pharmaceutical, toxicological, and so forth.

The SPC fulfils yet another communicative purpose. As stated by the European Commission in the 'Guideline on Summary of Product Characteristics' (1999), the SPC is the basis of information for health professionals on how to use the medicinal product safely and effectively.

With regard to content and structure (see figure 2.11 below), they are well defined by the Enterprise and Industry Directorate of the European Commission. As we have seen in figure 2.9 above, SPC contents derive directly from those contained in core data sheets. In turn, SPCs give rise to PILs.

---

1. TRADE NAME OF THE MEDICINAL PRODUCT
2. QUALITATIVE AND QUANTITATIVE COMPOSITION
3. PHARMACEUTICAL FORM
4. CLINICAL PARTICULARS
    4.1 Therapeutic indications
    4.2 Posology and method of administration
    4.3 Contra-indications
    4.4 Special warnings and special precautions for use
    4.5 Interaction with other medicaments and other forms of interaction
    4.6 Pregnancy and lactation
    4.7 Effects on ability to drive and use machines
    4.8 Undesirable effects
    4.9 Overdose
5. PHARMACOLOGICAL PROPERTIES
    5.1 Pharmacodynamic properties
    5.2 Pharmacokinetic properties
    5.3 Preclinical safety data
6. PHARMACEUTICAL PARTICULARS
    6.1 List of excipient(s)
    6.2 Incompatibilities
    6.3 Shelf-life
    6.4 Special precautions for storage
    6.5 Nature and contents of container

6.6 Instructions for use/handling
7. MARKETING AUTHORIZATION HOLDER
8. MARKETING AUTHORIZATION NUMBER
9. DATE OF FIRST AUTHORIZATION/RENEWAL OF AUTHORI-
   ZATION
10. DATE OF (PARTIAL) REVISION OF THE TEXT

---

*Figure 2.13. Structure of Summary of Product
Characteristics (EMEA)*

The above mentioned guide on the SPC specifies some norms that are useful for the translator, such as:

- International non-proprietary names (INN) should be used.
- The use of decimal points should be avoided where these can easily be removed.
- For safety reasons, micrograms should be always spelled in full.
- The pharmaceutical form should be described by the European Pharmacopoeia full standard term.
- The active substance should be referred to by its recommended INN, accompanied by its salt or hydrate form if relevant. If no INN exists, the European Pharmacopoeia name should be used or if the substance is not in the pharmacopoeia, the usual common name should be used. In the absence of a common name, the exact scientific designation should be given. Substances not having an exact scientific designation should be described by a statement of how and from what they were prepared.

Reading this guide is strongly recommended. It provides us with the norms and criteria that will enable us make better decisions in the translation process.

See examples of this genre

In the following link you will find examples of texts belonging to this genre. Read some of them so as to become familiar with their communicative purpose, structure, types of information contained in each part of the structure, phraseology, terminology, style, and tenor.

- <http://www.emea.eu.int> (in 20 European languages)

Task 6. Comparing PILs and SPCs

1) Go to <http://www.emea.eu.int/htms/human/epar/a-fepar.htm> and click on 'Abilify'. Look for this pdf somewhere else in EMEA's site if by the time you carry out this task 'Abilify' pdf has been moved from the above section.

2) Go to 'Product Information' and click on the 'u' under 'EN'. Now you have downloaded a pdf document on Abilify with the following sections on the left column: 'Package Leaflet'; 'Summary of Product Characteristics'; 'Manufacturing Authorization Holder'; 'Conditions of the Marketing Authorization'; and 'Labelling'.

3) Click on 'Package Leaflet' and go to page 107. Now you have the PIL of 'Abilify' 5 mg tablets. Read it carefully.

4) Now read the SPC of 'Abilify' 5 mg tablets between pages 2 and 10 of the same pdf document.

5) Compare these two genres and explore the differences between them using these questions: What information has been added in the PIL? What information has been omitted in the PIL? Are the headings for sections the same in both cases? How is specialized terminology presented? How are the readers addressed?

6) Go to <http://www.abilify.com>. Who are the main users of this website? What are its main aims? How many different genres can you identify in this website? Are all of them addressed to the same readership?

7) Find information about 'Abilify' (aripiprazole) in your target language which is distributed online for different purposes and readers, and therefore, distributed by means of different genres. Bear in mind what has been said in this chapter (see sub-section about PIL) about the different brand names and generic names of the same drug.

Case Report (CR)

The case report is arguably the oldest and most basic form of communication in medicine (Wildsmith, 2003: 85). Depending on the research journals where they are published, or the educational or clinical contexts in which they are produced and used, CRs are also known as 'clinical case reports', 'case studies', 'clinical case studies', 'clinical cases', or 'case histories'.

A case report is typically written by a clinician to describe and discuss an instance of a disease in a single patient. The communicative purpose of the CR is three-fold: 1) to share relevant clinical information with other clinicians and, therefore, help them improve their clinical practice; 2) to stimulate further research in a particular field or on a specific issue; and 3) to teach medical students how to approach complex clinical practice in an efficient way.

CRs normally describe or illustrate an aspect of the condition, the treatment, and adverse reactions to treatment. Have a look at the following example:

> H.L. is a 46 year old Afro-American female, with a past medical history significant for hypothyroidism and beta-thalassemia, who was otherwise healthy until two weeks prior to admission. At that time she noted onset of a sore throat, malaise and low-grade fevers. Four days prior to admission, she experienced fever to 104°F, chills, nausea and vomiting, and arthralgias and myalgias. She presented to the Johns Hopkins Bayview Medical.
> (Source: <http://www.hopkins-arthritis.som.jhmi.edu/case/case2/2_case.html>)

CRs are typically expository texts, that it, there is little or no argumentation or instruction. Facts are narrated and objects described so that the reader can easily form a mental image of them and understand them. They contain primary information, that is, hitherto unpublished material. In this sense, they contribute to scientific research by providing new, up-to-date information very rapidly. However, it is considered to be a weak type of research since it is supported by the evidence of just one single example.

The CR has its origins in medical teaching. In the 19th century, clinical teaching gradually shifted from lectures accounting for disease by theories and classifications more speculative than factually verified to bedside analysis of cases (Huth, 1999: 103). Helping the reader – a medical student or another clinician – to recognize and deal with a similar problem should one ever present itself in the future is of critical importance. Greenhalgh (2001: 52) provides a typical situation in which a case report can be needed to satisfy communicative needs:

> A doctor notices that two babies born in his hospital have absent limbs (phocomelia). Both mothers had taken a new drug (thalidomide) in early pregnancy. The doctor wishes to alert his colleagues worldwide to the possibility of drug related damages as quickly as possible.

Basically, the reader of a CR must have a clear understanding of: a) what happened to the patient; b) the sequence of events and the time scale involved; and c) why management followed the lines that it did (Wildsmith, 2003: 85).

Although different research journals have their own norms as far as structure and length of CRs, most published CRs have the following sections, the 'Case description' being the most important:

- Title
- Author(s)
- Introduction
- Background or literature review

- Case description
  - Case history
  - Examination
  - Intervention
- Outcome
- Discussion
- Summary

From the point of view of information flow, CRs may contain data from the patient's medical record that help the reader to understand the present condition. In turn, CRs directly or indirectly provide information to more systematic and sophisticated scientific work, such as:

- Case series: collections of similar case reports involving patients who were given similar treatment.
- Case control studies: studies in which patients who have a particular condition are compared with people who do not have it.
- Cohort studies: studies in which patients who currently have a certain condition and/or receive a particular treatment are followed over time and compared with another group who are not affected by the disease under investigation.
- Randomized controlled studies: studies in which there are two groups, a treatment group which receives the treatment under investigation, and a control group which receives either no treatment or some standard default treatment. Patients are randomly assigned to groups.
- Double blind studies: studies in which neither the patient nor the physician know whether the patient is receiving the treatment of interest or the control treatment.
- Systematic reviews: comprehensive surveys of a topic in which all the primary studies of the highest level of evidence undertaken by different research teams in different locations have been systematically identified, appraised, and then summarized in accordance with an explicit and reproducible methodology.
- Meta-analysis: surveys in which the results of all of the studies included are sufficiently similar statistically that the results are combined and analyzed as if they were one study.

For more information on these genres and sub-genres, go to <http://library.downstate.edu/EBM2>.

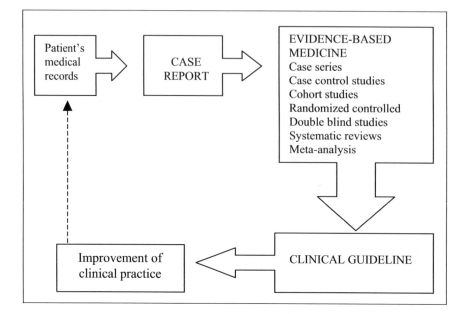

Figure 2.14. System of genres: research and its transference
to clinical practice

See examples of this genre

In the following links you will find examples of texts belonging to this genre. Read some of them so as to become familiar with their communicative purpose, structure, types of information contained in each part of the structure, phraseology, terminology, style, and tenor.

- <http://info.med.yale.edu/labmed/casestudies/casestudy.html>
- <http://www.crcpr-online.com/>
- <http://www.indiana.edu/~m555/cases/cases.html>
- <http://www.mic.ki.se/MEDCASES.html#A07>
- <http://ccs.sagepub.com/>
- <http://www.kcom.edu/faculty/chamberlain/cases.htm>

Clinical Guidelines (CG)

Although much biomedical research is carried out to improve clinical practice, not all of it is equally relevant. Besides clinicians simply don't have access to all documents nor the time to read the huge amounts of research literature that are generated and published every week in order to extract the knowledge needed to improve their own clinical practice. Clinical guidelines are meant to transfer relevant biomedical research to the clinic (see figure 2.14). Thus, clinical guidelines – also known as 'clinical practice guidelines' and 'practice guidelines' – are systematically developed statements to assist practitioner and patient decisions about appropriate health care for specific clinical circumstances. They offer concise instruction on clinical practice and can be developed at a national or local level by multidisciplinary groups. Thus, CGs are documents written by teams of experts for experts and are usually developed by multidisciplinary groups of researchers and addressed to practitioners. Their main purpose is to make explicit recommendations designed to influence what clinicians do. In addition, CGs are used to standardize and raise the quality of medical care, and to reduce several kinds of risk – to the patient, to the healthcare provider, to medical insurers and health plans.

Depending on the methodology used for developing them, several types of CGs can be distinguished: expert-opinion-based guidelines, consensus-based guidelines and evidence-based guidelines. The latter are based on a thorough evaluation of evidence and are defined as the way a procedure is done or a condition is managed. They have been developed in the context of evidence-based medicine and evidence-based health care. Evidence-based medicine is the conscientious, explicit and judicious use of current evidence in making decisions about the care of individual patients. The practice of evidence-based medicine and health care requires the integration of individual clinical expertise with the best available external clinical evidence from systematic research.

Although the writing of CGs is not regulated by strict norms, there are several legal instruments both at national and supranational levels. For instance, Recommendation Rec(2001)13, adopted by the Committee of Ministers of the Council of Europe on 10 October 2001 set up under the authority of the European Health Committee and developed by the Committee of Experts on Developing a Methodology Guidelines on Best Medical Practices, is intended to establish a framework for drawing up clinical practice guidelines in EU member states, and harmonize the national and international methodology of translating the best available evidence into the best medical practice.

There are other standardization bodies with a wider reach. The Guidelines International Network is an international non-profit-making association of organizations and individuals involved in clinical practice guidelines. Founded in November 2002, G-I-N has now 67 organizational members and partners representing 34 countries from North and South America, Asia, Europe and Oceania, plus the WHO. G-I-N seeks to improve the quality of health care by promoting systematic development of clinical practice guidelines and their application into practice, through supporting international collaboration.

There is also an international project for appraising clinical guidelines: the AGREE Collaboration. This project has developed an appraisal instrument to assess clinical guidelines and to harmonize guideline development through established networks. The purpose of the Appraisal of Guidelines Research & Evaluation (AGREE) Instrument is to provide a framework for assessing the quality of clinical practice guidelines. The AGREE Instrument assesses both the quality of the reporting, and the quality of some aspects of recommendations. AGREE instruments provides translations in 14 languages (Bosnian, Danish, Dutch, English, Finnish, French, German, Greek, Italian, Norwegian, Portuguese, Russian, Spanish, Swedish) can be consulted at:<http://www.agreecollaboration. org/translations>.

See examples of this genre

In the following links you will find examples of texts belonging to this genre. Read some of them so as to become familiar with their communicative purpose, structure, types of information contained in each part of the structure, phraseology, terminology, style, and tenor.

- <http://www.escardio.org/knowledge/guidelines>
- <http://www.eguidelines.co.uk>
- <http://www.sign.ac.uk/guidelines/published/index.html>
- <http://www.fisterra.com/guias2/no_explor/categorias.asp>
- <http://www.acc.org/clinical/statements.htm>
- <http://mdm.ca/cpgsnew/cpgs/index.asp>
- <http://medicine.ucsf.edu/resources/guidelines>

Clinical Trial Protocol (CTP)

Let's have a look at the following real communicative situation. Many women of a certain age, who, among other things, have a family history of breast cancer or who have had a number of breast biopsies, are thought to be at increased risk of developing the disease. The Clinical Trial Group (CTG) of the National Cancer Institute of Canada (NCIC) and the Grupo Español de Investigación en Cáncer de Mama (GEICAM) are promoting a study of a new drug in Canada, the United States and Spain to determine whether and to what extent it reduces the incidence of breast cancer in such women. This type of investigation is called a clinical trial and requires a document – a clinical trial protocol – in which all relevant aspects of the investigation are reflected and properly stored for further communicative uses, such as requesting marketing authorization.

Thus, clinical trials – also called 'clinical studies' – are experiments performed on human subjects in order to describe the pharmacological and pharmacodynamic effects of products, any adverse reactions as well as any other matters related to their safety and efficacy. A clinical trial protocol is a document that describes the objectives, purpose, and design of the trial, the selection and treatment of subjects, statistical considerations, and other issues related to the methodology and organization of the study. It can be written by a chief researcher in the case of multicentre trials, when trials are carried out in more than one centre, as in the example above, or by a principal researcher for single centre trials.

A CTP must be submitted to the appropriate authorities when requesting authorization for a clinical trial of a medicinal product for human use. It is attached to the application form, along with the researcher's brochure, and other medically-related research data, such as the medicinal research product dossier, or the summary of product characteristics for products with a marketing authorization in the EU.

In the European Union, the United States of America and Japan, content and macrostructure of CTPs are regulated by the Good Clinical Practice (GCP) standards, issued by the International Conference on Harmonization of Technical Requirements for Registration of Pharmaceuticals for Human Use (IHC). Authorities in Canada and Australia also comply with these guidelines. In addition, CTPs are regulated in the European Union by Directive 2001/20/CE.

Moreover, protocols are regulated in the European Union by Directive 2001/20/CE. There are some documents relating to this Directive:

- Detailed guidance for the request for authorization of a clinical trial on a medicinal product for human use to the competent authorities, notification of substantial amendments and declaration of the end of the trial (18/10/2005)
- Detailed guidance on the application format and documentation to be submitted in an application for an Ethics Committee opinion on the clinical trial on medicinal products for human use (26/04/2004)
- Detailed guidance on the collection, verification and presentation of adverse reaction reports arising from clinical trials on medicinal products for human use (26/04/2004)
- Detailed guidance on the European clinical trials database (EUDRACT Database) (26/04/2004)
- Detailed guidance on the European database of Suspected Unexpected Serious Adverse Reactions (Eudravigilance – Clinical Trial Module) (26/04/2004)
- Question and answer document for clinical trials (25/01/2005)
- Note for guidance on Good Clinical Practice CMP/ICH/135/95

Individual states may also have additional regulations. This is the case, for instance, in Spain (Real Decreto 223/2004).

Terminology – abbreviations included – must be consistent with that used by the ICH or the regulatory organization in a particular country. Terms have to be used accurately, e.g. differences must be taken into account when referring to adverse event (AE), adverse drug reaction (ADR), serious adverse event (SAE) or serious adverse drug reaction (serious ADR). In order to facilitate this task, a glossary with commonly used terms is included in CPMP/ICH/135/95. This document also includes the structure of a protocol trial and common contents included in it:

- General Information
- Background Information
- Trial Objectives and Purpose
- Trial Design
- Selection and Withdrawal of Subjects
- Treatment of Subjects
- Assessment of Efficacy
- Assessment of Safety
- Statistics
- Direct Access to Source Data/Documents
- Quality Control and Quality Assurance
- Ethics
- Data Handling and Recordkeeping
- Financing and Insurance
- Publication Policy
- Supplements

See examples of this genre

In the following links you will find examples of texts belonging to this genre. Read some of them so as to become familiar with their communicative purpose, structure, types of information contained in each part of the structure, phraseology, terminology, style, and tenor.

- <http://www.roche-trials.com/index.html>
- <www.niaid.nih.gov/dmid/ clinresearch/protocol_template.doc>
- <www.ucl.ac.uk/biomed-r-d/guides/guide_asrprep_submission.doc>
- <www.ahc.umn.edu/img/assets/11663/2006_02_10_GCP_Protocol_Template_Final.doc>
- <glrce.org/~glrceadmincore/documents/NIH%20Clinial%20trial%20protocol%20template.doc>
- <http://www.cancer.gov/PREVENTION/CTR/consortia/Step1-ProtoDev.html>
- <http://www.hc-sc.gc.ca/dhp-mps/prodpharma/applic-demande/guide-ld/clini/ctdcta_ctddec_e.html#3>

Task 7. Exploring national legislation in your country

1) Find the regulatory body for clinical trials in your country.
2) Find out about regulations for clinical trials in your country.
3) Which parts of the legislation may affect the task of the medical translator? How?

Review Article (RA)

Biomedical research generates a wealth of information every week. Researchers, physicians, general practitioners, and other health professionals as well as undergraduate and postgraduate students, constantly need to update their knowledge for different purposes: carrying out further research, improving clinical practice, developing new drugs, acquiring professional knowledge and skills and so forth. Review articles provide them with rigorous overviews of the most relevant research in a particular area so that they do not have to access, collect, select, read, and analyze the primary sources of biomedical research information − mainly original articles (see chapter 4 for more information on the original article as a research genre).

Thus the RA is a synoptic paper whose purpose is twofold: 'It spares clinicians the burden of searching and sifting the literature for reliable guidance in practice. It tells investigators where their research field stands on a particular problem and may suggest what directions new research should take' (Huth, 1999: 93).

Authors of RAs are experts at the cutting edge in their particular field. Their role as reviewers is that of a teacher who guides students through a sea of information. Reviewers have to be rigorous in their methodology and impartial in their assessment of the information.

Traditionally, reviews have relied mainly on the individual knowledge of the reviewer as an authority in a particular field, and have been written from a personal point of view, *ex cathedra*. However in areas in which there is a wealth of valuable information, and with the advent of evidence-based medicine, reviews have become far less *ex cathedra* and far more systematic and objective. A meta-analysis is a type of systematic review in which data from separate studies that address a similar research question are combined qualitatively and then analyzed statistically.

Although there is no fixed structure for review articles, most of them contain the following sections: a) introduction, in which the reviewer explains the question addressed, tries to convince readers that the article is worth reading, and demonstrates to them that it is informed and authoritative; b) methods, that is, a statement of how data were selected; c) body of the review, that is, the presentation of data; d) conclusion in which the initial question is answered.

Task 8. Exploring the structure of review articles

1) Go to the *British Medical Journal* website <http://wwwbmj.bmj-journals.com> and select three different review articles from different issues.

2) Read them carefully. Are they addressed to the same readership? Do they have the same aims? What are they? Do they have the same structure?

3) Go to the *New England Journal of Medicine* at <http://www.nejm.org> and to *The Lancet* at <http://www.thelancet.com>. Select a review article from each of the journals. Read them.

4) Compare the structure of the five articles and the type of information in each part of the structure. Are they the same?

5) Go the section about information for authors on the website of each of the three journals, and read what it says about review articles. Is there any significant difference between the three?

See examples of this genre

In the following links you will find examples of texts belonging to this genre. Read some of them so as to become familiar with their communicative purpose, structure, types of information contained in each part of the structure, phraseology, terminology, style, and tenor.

- <http://www.cochrane.org/index.htm>
- <http://www.freemedicaljournals.com> This site offers free access to online biomedical research journals in several languages where you can find review articles.

Standard Operating Procedure (SOP)

Every effective quality system is based on standard operating procedures. SOPs are written descriptions and instructions used in many professional practices to ensure the quality of products and processes and compliance with the current regulations and require consistency/uniformity in the performance of specific functions. They normally describe routine or repetitive tasks carried out by an organization – like a pharmaceutical laboratory, or a hospital – as well as procedures to be followed when responding to abnormal situations. The presence of these quality documents is essential when inspections take place since the most frequently reported deficiencies during inspections are the lack of written SOPs and/or the failure to adhere to them.

SOPs usually belong to a work plan or to a Quality Assurance Project Plan. They are written by experts who have a deep knowledge of the activities performed in the organization and of the organization's internal structure. These documents are addressed to the appropriate authorities (also Quality Audits) as well as to all those involved in the procedures described, providing them with the information they need to perform a task properly and improve consistency in the quality of products or outcomes. They can also be used to train new personnel. Thus, they are highly specialized, formal texts.

Standard Operating Procedures are regularly reviewed and updated to ensure that they encourage efficient working practices that comply with the ever increasing government regulatory framework that we have to operate within.

SOPs should be easy to read, expressed simply and concisely and the information provided should be unambiguous, explicit and not excessively complex. Terminology must be consistent with that used and recognized by those involved in the organization.

SOPs are usually divided into short sections and subsections and sometimes contain diagrams, flow charts and bullet points for ease of reading. Unlike SPCs, SOPs do not have one single template. The structure varies with each organization and with the type of procedure described. However, SOPs often include:

- A title page with a title identifying the procedure described, a SOP identification (ID) number, date of issue and/or revision, department or branch to which the SOP applies, and the signatures and signature dates of those who wrote and approved the SOP.
- A table of contents.
- Description of the procedure (purpose, applicable regulations, step-by-step description of the procedure).
- Attached documents.

In clinical research, SOPs are defined by the International Conference on Harmonization (ICH) as 'detailed, written instructions to achieve uniformity of the performance of a specific function'. SOPs are necessary for clinical research organizations – pharmaceutical companies, sponsors, contract research organizations or any other party involved in clinical research – to achieve maximum safety and efficiency of the performed clinical research operations. The SOPs cover all aspects of a clinical trial, including:

- Protocol preparation
- Ethical approval
- Assessing and monitoring trial sites
- Safety data reporting
- Checking data integrity

- Clinical report writing
- Database preparation
- Validating computer systems

Common problems when translating SOPs include references to the culture of the source text such as allusions to the country where the text has been written and to its regulations, to the name of a certain medicine – trade name, international non-proprietary name, United States Adopted Name, British Approved Name, Japanese Accepted Name – and to different units of measurement, e.g. international units of measurements vs imperial units.

Moreover, source texts are not as unequivocal and explicit as they should be, so translators sometimes have to struggle to produce a good target text. If the wording of any item of information is open to several interpretations, the translator must contact the organization or SOP writer in order to make the meaning absolutely clear; nothing must be left to the reader's imagination.

In the following links you will find examples of texts belonging to this genre. Read some of them so as to become familiar with their communicative purpose, structure, types of information contained in each part of the structure, phraseology, terminology, style, and tenor.

- <http://www.niaid.nih.gov/ncn/sop/adverseevents.htm>
- <http://www.emea.eu.int/pdfs/human/sop/SOP3043en.pdf>
- <http://www.emea.eu.int/pdfs/general/sop/SOP0001en.pdf>
- <http://www.emea.eu.int/pdfs/general/sop/SOP0025en.pdf>
- <http://wwwmcg.edu/Research/animal/rtf/SOPs.rtf>

Drug Advertisement (DA)

Health is one of the most important issues in society and the pharmaceutical industry, one of the most powerful economic sectors worldwide, makes money out of health – or the lack of it. After a new drug has been developed in the laboratory, tested in animals and humans, and approved by the appropriate authorities, pharmaceutical laboratories try to sell as much of it as they can. Marketing in its different forms is the tool laboratories – like any other company in any other economic sector – use to achieve their goals, and advertising, in particular, is one of the most important marketing strategies used by them to sell their products. Now let's have a look at the following text:

Every breath you take

Asthma is a growing problem in developed countries with 100-150 million people affected by this breathing disorder.

More than 20 years after a song called "Every breath you take" became a

---

> worldwide hit for The Police, the single remains one of the most popular on many radio stations' play lists.
>
> Originally, it was thought that it was a love song – the title was also used for a romantic novel by best-selling US author, Judith McNaught – but closer examination showed that the song was not a paean to passion.
>
> The title has also been used by several authors when describing their – or their loved ones – experiences with asthma. And, once again, the evocative title of these articles masks the profound effect that asthma can have on sufferers.
>
> Imagine for a moment what it would be like to find every single breath that you take requires an effort of monumental proportion. Imagine too being unable to climb a few stairs or lift a small child because you cannot get enough breath. This is how uncontrolled asthma can affect people's lives.
>
> (Source: <http://www.gsk.com/infocus/asthma.htm>)

If you read this and know someone who suffers from this affliction, you will probably want to know what treatments are available and where. Some drugs can be bought at the chemist's over the counter, while others can only be obtained with a doctor's prescription. The former are called "over the counter" drugs and the latter "prescription" drugs.

Task 9. Understanding drug advertisements

1) Go to the <http://www.gsk.com/infocus/asthma.htm> and read the whole article.
2) Translate the title into your mother tongue. Justify your translation.
3) Find out at the same site which drug is commercialized by this particular pharmaceutical laboratory to treat asthma.
4) Is it a prescription drug or an over-the-counter drug?
5) Find at the same site other texts used to promote the use of that particular drug.

Owing to possible drug-related health risks, the pharmaceutical industry is heavily regulated, not only as far as development and experimentation is concerned, but also in relation to the advertising and promotion of its products. For instance, in the EU Member States, advertising of medicinal products is subject to Title VIII of the European Parliament and the Council of the European Union Directive 2001/83/EC on the advertising of medicines for human use. In the United States, the Drug Marketing, Advertising, and Communications Divisions, the Food and Drug Administration (FDA) regulates all advertising and promotional activities for prescription drugs.

Over-the-counter drugs, on the other hand, can be advertised in the mass media (internet, television, radio, newspapers, magazines, and so forth) to the general public. However, their potential target recipient includes not only the consumers themselves – that is, the patients – but also physicians, pharmacists and other health professionals who may be in a position to recommend such drugs to patients.

Advertising prescription drugs to the general public is banned in the EU Member States. Article 88 of the Title VIII of Directive 2001/83/EC on the advertising of medicines for human use states: "1. Member States shall prohibit the advertising to the general public of medicinal products which: (a) are available on medical prescription only, in accordance with Title VI". Therefore, medical practitioners become a sort of bridge in the advertising process between the seller – the pharmaceutical laboratory – and the consumer – the patient in those countries where only over-the-counter drugs can be advertised in the mass media to the general public. So, how are prescription drugs advertised to medical practitioners?

Firstly, by means of advertisements placed in medical journals, on pharmaceutical companies' websites or other specialized biomedical websites which allow advertisements. Secondly, by pharmaceutical sales representatives, who, in addition to oral explanations and presentations, provide practitioners with brochures, clinical guidelines, leaflets information for patients, and samples of the product.

- Most pharmaceutical companies advertise medicinal products on their web sites. Look for two or three of them and find examples of texts belonging to this genre. Read some of them so as to become familiar with their communicative purpose, structure, types of information contained in each part of the structure, phraseology, terminology, style, and tenor.

2.6 Further tasks

Task 10. Becoming familiar with clinical guidelines

Find five clinical guidelines in your target language about five different diseases or conditions. Are they addressed to the same readership? Do they have the same structure?

Task 11. Exploring other genres

Choose other genres presented in chapter 1, but not developed further in this chapter, and explore them in the same way as we have done here: Who uses them? In which situations? For which purposes? What is their typical structure? Is there any legislation that regulates them? What kind of language and terminology is used in them?

2.7 Further reading

Bazerman, Charles (1998) 'Emerging perspectives on the many dimensions of scientific discourse', in J.R. Martin and Robert Veel (eds) *Reading Science. Critical and Functional Perspectives of Discourses of Science*, London and New York: Routledge, 15-30.

García, Isabel and Vicent Montalt (2002) 'Translating into Textual Genres', *Linguistica Antverpiensia* (Special Issue: *Linguistics and Translation Studies; Translation Studies and Linguistics*), Volume 1, Antwerp: Hoger Institute vor Vertalerse & Tolken, 135-143.

García, Isabel (ed.) (2005) *El género textual y la traducción. Reflexiones teóricas y aplicaciones pedagógicas*, Bern: Peter Lang.

Martin J.R. and Robert Veel (1998) (eds) *Reading Science. Critical and Functional Perspectives on Discourses of Science*, London and New York: Routledge.

Montalt, Vicent and Isabel García (2002) 'Multilingual Corpus-based Research of Medical Genres for Translation Purposes: The Medical Corpus of the GENTT project', in José Chabás, Joëlle Rey and Rolf Gaser (eds) *Proceedings of the 2nd Conference on Specialized Translation*, Barcelona: Universitat Pompeu Fabra, 299-306.

Vihla, Minna (1999) *Medical Writing. Modality in Focus*, Amsterdam, Atlanta: Rodopi. [Language and Computers: Studies in Practical Linguistics No 28].

On Fact Sheets for Patients

Albin, Veronica (1998) 'Translating and Formatting Medical Texts for Patients with Low Literacy Skills', in Henry Fischbach (ed.) *Translation and Medicine*, Amsterdam and Philadelphia: John Benjamins, 117-130.

Mayor Serrano, María Blanca (2005) 'Análisis contrastivo (inglés-español) de la clase de texto «folleto de salud» e implicaciones didácticas para la formación de traductores médicos', *Panace@ Revista de Medicina y Traducción* 6(20): 132-141. [Available at: http://www.medtrad.org/panacea]

On Informed Consents

'A Guide to Understanding Informed Consent' (National Cancer Institute, U.S.

National Institutes of Health) [Available at: http://www.cancer.gov/clinicaltrials/
    conducting/informed-consent-guide/page2]
'Informed Consent' (American Medical Association) [Available at: http://www.ama-
    assn.org/ama/pub/category/4608.html]
'Patient information sheet and consent form' (North Glasgow University Hospitals)
    [Available at: http://www.show.scot.nhs.uk/ngt/research/forms/Scottish_Exec_
    PIS_Guidelines_Feb01.html]

On Patient Information Leaflets

'A guideline on the readability of the label and package leaflet of medicinal products
    for human use', European Commission. [Available at: http://ec.europa.eu/enter-
    prise/pharmaceuticals/eudralex/vol-2/c/gl981002.pdf]
'Guidance documents', U.S. Food and Drug Administration Center for Drug Evalu-
    ation and Research. [Available at: http://www.fda.gov/cder/guidance/index.htm]
'Guidance on the User Testing of Patient Information Leaflets', MHRA, 2005.
    [Available at: http://www.mhra.gov.uk/home/groups/pl-a/documents/publication/
    con1004417.pdf]
'Labels and patient information leaflets for medicines', MHRA. [Available at: http://
    www.mhra.gov.uk/home/idcplg?IdcService=SS_GET_PAGE&nodeId=164]
'Notice to applicants: Guideline on the packaging information of medicinal products
    for human use authorised by the Community', European Commission. [Available
    at: http://ec.europa.eu/enterprise/pharmaceuticals/eudralex/vol-2/c/bluebox_03_
    2005.pdf]

On Summaries of Product Characteristics

'A Guideline of Summary of Product Characteristics', Enterprise and Industry
    Directorate-General, European Commission, 2005. [Available at: http://pharmacos.
    eudra.org/F2/eudralex/vol-2/C/SPCGuidRev1-Oct2005.pdf]

On Case Reports

Huth, Edward J. (1999) 'The Case Report and the Case-Series Analysis', in Edward
    J. Huth *Writing and Publishing in Medicine*, 3rd ed. Baltimore: Williams &
    Wilkins, 103-110.
'Researching and Writing a Case Report'. [Available at: http://www.lib.uwaterloo.
    ca/discipline/opt/opt.html#top]
Wildsmith, J. (2003) 'How to write a case report', in G.M. Hall (ed.) *How to Write a
    Paper*, London, British Medical Journal Books, 85-91.

On Clinical Guidelines

The AGREE Collaboration (2001) *Appraisal of Guidelines for Research & Evaluation (AGREE) Instrument*; [Available at: www.agreecollaboration.org]

The European Health Committee (CDSP) (2002) 'Developing a Methodology for Drawing up Guidelines on Best Medical Practices Recommendation". Rec (2001)13 adopted by the Committee of Ministers of the Council of Europe on 10 October 2001 and explanatory memorandum; Strasbourg: Council of Europe Publishing. [Available at: http://www.aezq.de/aezq/kooperationspartner_en/pdf/europaratmeth.pdf]

World Health Organization 'Guidelines for WHO Guidelines', Global Programme on Evidence for Health Policy. 10 March 2003. [Available at: http://whqlibdoc.who.int/hq/2003/EIP_GPE_EQC_2003_1.pdf]

On Clinical Trial Protocols

'Detailed guidance for the request for authorisation of a clinical trial on a medicinal product for human use to the competent authorities, notification of substantial amendments and declaration of the end of the trial'. [Available at: http://dg3.eudra.org/F2/pharmacos/docs/Doc2005/10_05/CA_14-2005.pdf]

'Directive 2001/20/EC of the European Parliament and of the Council'. [Available at: http://eudract.emea.eu.int/docs/Dir2001-20_en.pdf]

'Guide to Protocol Content and Format to Meet ICH GCP Standards'. [Available at: http://www.ucl.ac.uk/biomed-r-d/guides/guide_protocol_content_%20format.doc]

'Note for Guidance on Good Clinical Practice' (CPMP/ICH/135/95). [Available at: http://www.emea.eu.int/pdfs/human/ich/013595en.pdf]

On Review Articles

Forgacs, Ian (2003) '12: How to Write a Review', in G.M. Hall (ed.) *How to Write a Paper*, London, British Medical Journal Books, 92-98.

Greenhalgh, Trisha (2001) 'Chapter 8: Papers that summarize other papers (systematic reviews and meta-analysis)', in *How to Read a Paper*, London: British Medical Journal Books, 120-138.

http://authors.nejm.org/Misc/Articles.asp
http://bmj.bmjjournals.com/advice/sections.shtml
http://www.cebm.utoronto.ca/glossary/index.htm#sr
http://www.thelancet.com/authors/lancet/authorinfo

On Standard Operating Procedures

Fries, Ruth Ann (2002) 'Standard operating procedures for clinical research coordinators', *Drug Information Journal*, Apr-Jun 2002. [Available at: http://www.looksmartscience.com/p/articles/mi_qa3899/is_200204/ai_n9057342].

'Helping to achieve a high level of proficiency, production, and safety'. [Available at: http://pubs.acs.org/hotartcl/chas/98/julaug/stan.html].

Jones, Anne Catesby (2004) 'Translating SOPs in a Pharmaceutical Manufacturing Environment', *Translation Journal* 8(2). [Available at: http://accurapid.com/journal/28biomeda.htm].

3. Understanding the content of the source text

> [...] a lack of formal medical training is not necessarily an insurmountable obstacle to the budding medical translator. What is essential is not a medical degree, but a broad understanding of the fundamentals and knowledge of how to acquire, in the most efficient manner, an understanding of other elements as and when necessary.
>
> Judy Wakabayashi (1996: 357)

Overview of chapter

We understand the source text so that we can make the target reader understand the target text. Understanding the mechanisms of text comprehension (3.1) has a two-fold purpose: a) to become aware of how we process the content of the source text; b) to grasp how our readers process the content of the target text. A medical degree provides the medical knowledge and skills needed to start a career as a health professional. Medical translators do not necessarily need a medical degree because we do not need the active knowledge and skills to carry out tasks in the clinic or in the laboratory, such as diagnosing, prescribing, operating, curing, and so forth. What is useful, however, is to acquire some background medical knowledge in order to be able to understand source texts properly (3.2). Developing comprehension strategies such as text mapping, using etymological information, exploring metaphors, or paraphrasing implicit information (3.3) can enhance our ability to understand medical texts and our sense of security when dealing with topics with which we are not familiar.

3.1 How we understand texts

This may sound very obvious but it is worth remembering in the context of medical translation: if we don't understand the source text, we can't translate it. As translators, one of our basic tasks is to understand so that we can enable our readers to understand the same. Whatever we fail to understand in the source text is likely to be either misinterpreted or not understood at all by the reader of the target text.

Although this is not the right occasion to review it, it is worth mentioning that there is a wealth of scientific literature on the cognitive mechanisms involved in text comprehension – here we draw mainly on Kintsch (1998), Jackendoff (1983), Wilson (1994) and Brown (1994) – from which the following conclusions can be drawn:

- The text is like an iceberg: on the surface we only see part of it, which means that we often need to infer the underlying intended meaning.

- We use information from the text itself, from the context and from the previous knowledge that we have about the topic of the text in order to infer the intended meaning.
- In the process of understanding a text, we construct a mental representation of it from the words on the page but also from personal perceptions of reality, ideas, images, and even emotions.
- These elements may come from a variety of sources: perceptual systems, memories, knowledge, beliefs, body states, or goals when reading.
- Comprehension occurs when the cognitive elements that enter into the process are meaningfully related to one another.
- The cognitive elements that do not fit the pattern of the majority are suppressed from the mental representation.
- A reader has specific goals for understanding a text, in our case, translating it into a different language so that the target reader can understand it too.
- A comprehender has a given background of knowledge and experience of the topic of the text. In the case of medical translators without a medical degree, this background knowledge has to be acquired gradually through other means.
- A comprehender is in a given perceptual situation, in our case, receiving information input only from the printed words on a page of text.
- From these words, the reader constructs basic idea units in the form of propositions.
- Given these idea units in the form of propositions as well as the reader's goals, associated elements from her/his long-term memory (knowledge, experience) are retrieved to form an interrelated network with the already existing perceptual elements.
- Without the reader's long term memory (knowledge, experience) it is impossible to form the interrelated network and the mental representation of the text. Hence the importance of acquiring background medical knowledge (see section 3.2)
- The linguistic form of a sentence or expression can lead to more than one interpretation.
- Surrounding text and context are required to choose the appropriate interpretation and reject other interpretations which may be linguistically defensible.
- The closer the new information is connected with the surrounding text and context, the more relevant the interpretation.
- In the process of understanding a text we constantly make predictions or hypotheses that we either reinforce or reject in accordance with the information provided by the text.
- Source text authors are not omniscient and therefore are not always able to provide the reader with the optimum linguistic elements that would convey

the intended meaning clearly and economically. Medical translators may have to supply these for the reader.

- In the case of genre shifts (see 4.6), target readers may not have the same previous knowledge about the topic of the text as the source readers and may need extra information.

What's your comprehension style?

Wade (1990, as cited by Herrell and Jordan: 2002: 256-257) establishes general categories of comprehension styles according to their use of predictions and self-monitoring. You should be aware of them and decide which fits your comprehension style better. There may be more than one that reflects your behaviour as a comprehender depending on the complexity of the text you're dealing with and the degree of familiarity you have with its content.

- Good comprehenders interact with the text, constructing meanings and monitoring their own understanding.
- Non-risk takers rely heavily on the text and fail to go beyond the words on the page to make predictions, draw inferences or make connections.
- Non-integrators draw on clues from the text and also from past experience but don't integrate them.
- Schema imposers make an initial prediction or hypothesis and then try to make the meaning of the text fit that first impression.
- Storytellers are extremely dependent on prior knowledge and experiences. Rather than answering questions related to the information in the text, storytellers relate the questions to their own experiences.

Your aim as a medical translator should be the first one in the list above – good comprehenders – for which a series of habits that efficient readers generally employ to construct meaning are needed (Herrell and Jordan, 2000: 256):

- They read the text until they find out enough to formulate a hypothesis. (In other words, don't reach for the dictionary the first time you see a term you don't understand.)
- They evaluate the information they are reading and decide whether or not it fits their original hypothesis. (Thus, formulating hypotheses and evaluating them enables you to find the relevance of what you are reading.)
- They begin to make predictions about what will come next in the text and begin to make a series of predictions that are subsequently confirmed or modified according to the information they are reading. (Don't worry if your

predictions are not right. What really matters is that you make them and use them.)

- If their predictions are not confirmed, good readers self-monitor and use strategies to determine whether or not their past experiences, predictions, and overall understanding of the reading are making sense. (The more unfamiliar you are with the topic of the text, the more you should check that whatever you read does make sense.)

3.2 Background medical knowledge

This section provides an overview of the background medical knowledge you should acquire at this initial stage of your training, but does not provide the actual information itself: that is far beyond the scope of this book. Links are given so that you can read full texts and study the different body systems following the overviews provided in the table for each of these. Thus this section is conceived as a self-study starting point for the medical translator without a medical degree. For ease of reading and understanding this section is based on body systems and combines different types of information starting from the fundamental aspects of anatomy and physiology – the healthy person – and moving to pathology, diagnosis, and therapy – the sick person. We will follow the structure proposed by Gylys and Wedding (2005) in *Medical Terminology Systems. A Body System Approach*.

Integumentary system

The integument – from Latin 'integumentum' meaning cover – is the covering that separates the body from the environment. This covering protects the body's internal living tissues and organs against invasion by infectious organisms, and against dehydration and abrupt changes of temperature. It also acts as a receptor for touch, pressure, pain, heat and cold thus enabling communication with the environment. Finally the integumentary system helps dispose of waste materials and stores water, fat, and vitamin D. The integumentary system consists of the skin and its epidermal structures (integumentary glands, hair, and nails).

Anatomy and Physiology	Generalized diseases	Main diagnostic and therapeutic procedures	Main types of drugs
Epidermis, dermis, sebaceous glands, sweat glands, hair, nails.	Dermatitis, psoriasis, burns, skin cancer.	Intradermal test, patch test, scratch test, biopsy. Debridement, dermabrasion, fulguration, chemical peel, cryosurgery, incision and drainage.	Antifungals, antihistamines, antiseptics, corticosteroid anti-inflammatories, keratolytics, parasiticides, protectives.

A note on tasks 1 to 10

Links for all the tasks in the rest of this section can be found at the end of the chapter. In all the tasks, use any other information source you consider necessary (see chapter 6). Images of all kinds (photographs, drawings, animations, videos, etc.) are particularly useful. Avoid simply translating the texts you read. Make sure that everything you write makes sense.

Task 1. Understanding anatomical parts I

Explain in as much detail as possible the following notions in your target language focusing on structure and function: 'sudoriferous glands' and 'sebaceous glands'.

Digestive system

Food undergoes three processes in the human body. Once we ingest it, we digest it first by chewing it (mechanical digestion) and then by churning and mixing actions in the stomach (chemical digestion), thus breaking down food into smaller molecules that can be absorbed and used by the cells (absorption). Finally the molecules that cannot be digested or absorbed are eliminated from the body (elimination) through the anus in the form of faeces.

Anatomy and Physiology	Generalized diseases	Main diagnostic and therapeutic procedures	Main types of drugs
Mouth, pharynx, oesophagus, stomach, small intestine, large intestine, liver, pancreas, gallbladder.	Peptic ulcer disease, ulcerative colitis, bowel obstruction, haemorrhoids, liver disorders, diverticulitis, cancer.	Endoscopy, hepatitis panel, liver function tests, serum bilirubin, stool culture, cholecystography, computed tomography scan, ultrasonography, biopsy. Nasogastric intubation, anastomosis, colostomy, lithotripsy.	Antacids, antidiarrhoeals, anti-emetics, antispasmodics, laxatives.

Task 2. Understanding diseases I

Explain in as much detail as possible the following notions in your target language focusing on causes and effects: 'peptic ulcer disease' (PUD) and 'hepatitis A'.

Respiratory system

The lungs are the main organ of the respiratory system. Before the air reaches them, it passes through a number of other organs, such as the nose, the pharynx, the larynx, and the trachea. The main function of the respiratory system is to inhale oxygen, which is done in the first place through the nose, where the temperature and moisture content of the air are regulated. Another function of the nose is to filter out of the air impurities that might damage the lungs. Then the air goes down through the pharynx to the larynx and the trachea, which diverges into the right and the left bronchi. The bronchi further branch into secondary bronchi, bronchioles and alveoli. The lungs are formed by millions of alveoli and blood capillaries whose function is to exchange oxygen and carbon dioxide by means of inhalation and exhalation.

Anatomy and Physiology	Generalized diseases	Main diagnostic and therapeutic procedures	Main types of drugs
Upper respiratory tract, lower respiratory tract.	Asthma, chronic bronchitis, emphysema, influenza, pleural effusions, tuberculosis, pneumonia, cystic fibrosis, cancer.	Oximetry, polysomnography, spirometry, bronchoscopy, laryngoscopy, sputum culture, throat culture, chest radiography, lung scan. Aerosol therapy, lavage, postural drainage, rhinoplasty, pleurectomy, pneumectomy, thoracentesis.	Antihistamines, antitussives, bronchodilators, corticosteroids, decongestants, expectorants.

Task 3. Understanding diagnostic procedures I

Explain in as much detail as possible the following notions in your target language focusing on purpose, equipment, measurements, and steps of the procedure: 'oximetry' and 'bronchoscopy'.

Cardiovascular system

The main functions of the cardiovascular system are to circulate oxygen in the body, to remove carbon dioxide, and to provide cells with the nutrients they need to carry out their tasks. In addition, the cardiovascular system removes waste products from the metabolism to the excretory organs for disposal, protects the body against disease and infection, transports hormones, and regulates body temperature. Clotting stops bleeding after injury.

Anatomy and Physiology	Generalized diseases	Main diagnostic and therapeutic procedures	Main types of drugs
Arteries, capillaries, veins, heart, blood pressure.	Arteriosclerosis, coronary artery disease, endocarditis, varicose veins, cancer.	Cardiac catheterization, electrocardiogram, aortography, coronary angiography, echocardiography, venography. Cardioversion, embolization, angioplasty, atherectomy, phlebotomy, thrombolysis.	Antiarrhythmics, beta blockers, calcium channel blockers, diuretics, statins, nitrates, peripheral vasodilators.

Task 4. Understanding therapeutic procedures I

Explain in as much detail as possible the following notions in your target language focusing on purpose, equipment, measurements, and steps of the procedure: 'angioplasty' and 'thrombolysis'.

Blood, lymph, and immune systems

Blood is connective tissue made of a liquid medium called plasma and solid components suspended in it, mainly red and white blood cells and platelets. The most important functions of blood are to carry oxygen and nutrients to the body tissues, to remove carbon dioxide and other wastes, to provide defence against invasion by foreign substances, and to repair damaged tissue. The lymphatic system is made up of a fluid agent called lymph and a number of structures such as nodes, spleen, thymus, tonsils, and a network of lymph vessels. Lymph transports nutrients to the cells and collects waste products. The immune system protects the organism from outside biological influences by means of monocytes and lymphocytes. Thus the blood, lymph, and immune systems share the critical function of protecting the body against disease-causing agents.

Anatomy and physiology	Generalized diseases	Main diagnostic and therapeutic procedures	Main types of drugs
Blood: erythrocytes, leukocytes, platelets, plasma; Lymph system: lymph, lymph vessels, spleen, thymus, tonsils; Immune system: monocytes, lymphocytes.	Anaemias, AIDS, allergy, autoimmune disease, oedema, haemophilia, infectious mononucleosis, leukaemia, Hodgkin's disease, Kaposi's sarcoma.	Blood culture, complete blood count, differential count, haematocrit, lymphadenography, lymphangiography, bone marrow aspiration, bone marrow biopsy. Lymphangiectomy, transfusion, bone marrow transplantation.	Anticoagulants, antineoplastics, antiprotozoals, antivirals, fat-soluble vitamins, haemostatics, thrombolytics.

Task 5. Understanding types of drugs I

Explain in as much detail as possible the following notions in your target language focusing on their purposes and mechanisms of action: 'anticoagulants' and 'thrombolytics'. Provide some examples of specific anticoagulants and thrombolytics in your target language both in non-proprietary names and in commercial names.

Musculoskeletal system

Bones provide the framework of the body. Their main functions are to protect the internal organs such as the brain, the heart, or the lungs; to store calcium and other minerals; to produce blood cells within bone marrow; and to contribute to movement. Muscles are tissue composed of contractile cells. Their main function is to enable movement such as walking, talking, passage and elimination of food, propulsion of blood, and contraction of the bladder. In addition, they produce body heat, contribute to posture, and protect internal organs.

Anatomy and Physiology	Generalized diseases	Diagnostic and therapeutic procedures	Types of drugs
Muscles: skeletal, cardiac, and smooth. Bones: short, irregular, flat, and long.	Fractures, herniation, osteomyelitis, osteoporosis, scoliosis, kyphosis, lordosis, rheumatoid arthritis, muscular dystrophy, cancer.	Arthrography, computed tomography scan, discography, myelography. Amputation, anthrocentesis, arthroclasia, arthroscopy, bursectomy, bone grafting, synovectomy.	Opioid analgesics, salicylates, skeletal muscle relaxants.

Task 6. Understanding anatomical parts II

Explain in as much detail as possible the following notions in your target language focusing on structure and function: 'sternocleidomastoid' and 'intervertebral disk'.

Genitourinary system

The urinary system is composed of two kidneys, two ureters, the urinary bladder, two sphincter muscles, the prostate, and the urethra. It produces, stores, and carries urine. Its main purpose is to regulate extracellular fluids, such as plasma, tissue fluid, and lymph, by removing harmful substances, nitrogenous wastes, and excess of sodium, potassium and calcium, from plasma while retaining useful ones.

The male reproductive system's main purpose is to produce, maintain, and transport sperm. Sperm is produced in the seminiferous tubules of the testes, two organs contained in the scrotum. The testes also produce the male hormone testosterone, which is essential for the development of sperm.

Anatomy and Physiology	Generalized diseases	Diagnostic and therapeutic procedures	Types of drugs
Urinary system:	Pyelonephritis, glomerulonephritis,	Digital rectal examination,	Antibiotics, antidiuretics,

kidneys, ureters, bladder, urethra. Male reproductive system: testes, scrotum, epididymis, vas deferens, seminal vesicle, prostate gland, penis, urethra.	nephrolithiasis, bladder neck obstruction, benign prostatic hyperplasia, cryptorchidism, acute tubular necrosis, carcinoma of the prostate.	electromyography, testicular self-examination, cystoscopy, nephroscopy, urethroscopy, blood urea nitrogen (BUN), semen analysis, cystography, cystourethrography, pyelography. Haemodialysis, lithotripsy, circumcision, nephroplexy, orchidectomy, resection of the prostate, urethrotomy.	antispasmodics, diuretics, potassium supplements, androgens, anti-impotence agents, spermicides.

Task 7. Understanding diseases II

Explain in as much detail as possible the following notions in your target language focusing on causes and effects: 'nephrolithiasis' and 'carcinoma of the prostate'.

Female reproductive system

The female reproductive system is composed of internal organs (ovaries, fallopian tubes, uterus, vagina) and external genitalia (labia minora, labia majora, clitoris, and Bartholin glands). Their main functions are to produce female reproductive cells (ova), transport them to the site of fertilization, provide a favourable environment for a developing foetus, and produce female sex hormones. Ova are produced in the ovaries, two small organs set in the pelvic cavity below and to either side of the navel. After an ovum matures, it passes into the uterine tube. If sperm is present, fertilization occurs within the tube. The ovum, either fertilized or unfertilized, then passes down the fallopian tube, and into the womb, or uterus.

Anatomy and Physiology	Generalized diseases	Diagnostic and therapeutic procedures	Types of drugs
Female reproductive organs: ovaries, fallopian tubes, uterus and vagina; Mammary glands, menstrual cycle, pregnancy, labour, childbirth, menopause.	Menstrual disorders, endometriosis, vaginitis, gonorrhoea, syphilis, chlamydia, genital herpes, genital warts, trichomoniasis, breast cancer, cervical cancer.	Amniocentesis, colposcopy, laparoscopy, endometrial biopsy, mammography, pelvic ultrasonography, hysterosalpingography. Cerclage, caesarean birth, colpocleisis, cordocentesis, dilatation & curettage (D&C), episiorrhaphy, episiotomy, hysterectomy.	Antifungals, estrogens, oral contraceptives, oxytocics, prostaglandins.

Task 8. Understanding diagnostic procedures II

Explain in as much detail as possible the following notions in your target language focusing on purpose, equipment, measurements, and steps of the procedure: 'colposcopy' and 'mammography'.

Endocrine system

The endocrine system is responsible for maintaining a stable internal environment in the human body by producing chemical substances called hormones. It includes a number of endocrine glands (pituitary, thyroid, parathyroid, adrenal) that release the hormones necessary to regulate body functions. Hormones do not pass through tubes or ducts. They are secreted directly into the internal environment, where they are transmitted via the bloodstream or by diffusion and act on the metabolism of cells at distant points in the body.

Anatomy and Physiology	Generalized diseases	Diagnostic and therapeutic procedures	Types of drugs
Pituitary gland,	Graves' disease, toxic goitre,	Exophthalmometry, fasting blood	Insulins, oral antidiabetics,

thyroid gland, parathyroid glands, pancreas, pineal gland.	hypoparathyroidism, hyperparathyroidism, Addison's disease, Cushing's syndrome, diabetes, adenocarcinoma.	glucose (FBG), glucose tolerance test (GTT), insulin tolerance test, thyroid function test (TFT), radioactive iodine uptake (RAIU), thyroid scan. Parathyroidectomy, pinealectomy, thymectomy, thyroidectomy.	antithyroids, corticosteroids, growth hormone replacements, thyroid supplements.

Task 9. Understanding therapeutic procedures II

Explain in as much detail as possible the following notions in your target language focusing on purpose, equipment, measurements, and steps of the procedure: 'pinealectomy' and 'thyroidectomy'.

Nervous system

The nervous system is a network of specialized tissue that controls actions and reactions of the body and its adjustment to the environment. It consists of the central nervous system (brain and spinal cord) and the peripheral nervous systems, which is in its turn subdivided into two specialized systems: the somatic nervous system and the autonomic nervous system. The nervous system is built up of approximately 200 billion nerve cells, called neurons, half of which are found in the brain. When a neuron is chemically stimulated, it generates an impulse that passes from one neuron to another and carries information throughout the nervous system. Activities like walking and reasoning are regulated by the central nervous system, whereas the autonomic nervous system is a subsidiary system that regulates the iris of the eye and the action of the heart, blood vessels, glands, lungs, stomach, colon, bladder, and other visceral organs not subject to wilful control.

Anatomy and Physiology	Generalized diseases	Diagnostic and therapeutic procedures	Types of drugs
Neurons;	Bell's palsy,	Electroencephalography,	Analgesics,
neuroglia; central nervous system: brain, spinal cord, meninges; peripheral nervous system: cranial nerves, spinal nerves, somatic nervous system, autonomic nervous system.	ischaemic stroke, intracerebral haemorrhage, subarachnoid haemorrhage, epilepsy, Parkinson's disease, multiple sclerosis, Alzheimer's disease, psychosis, neurosis.	electromyography, lumbar puncture, magnetoencephalography (MEG), nerve conduction velocity (NCV), cerebrospinal fluid (CSF) analysis, angiography, myelography, brain scan, echoencephalography. Cryosurgery, stereotactic radiosurgery, thalomotomy, tractotomy, trephination, vagotomy.	anaesthetics, anticonvulsants, antiparkinsonian agents, hypnotics, antipsychotics, antidepressants, psychostimulants.

Task 10. Understanding types of drugs II

Explain in as much detail as possible the following notions in your target language focusing on their purposes and mechanisms of action: 'anaesthetics' and 'antidepressants'. Provide some examples of specific anaesthetics and antidepressants in your context both in non-proprietary names and in commercial names.

3.3 Developing text comprehension strategies

In medical translation text comprehension is often a non-linear, complex process. Only when we are very familiar with the topic and the genre of the text, can we read it and produce a translation straightaway sentence by sentence. Otherwise, in order to understand the source text properly we need to work through it in a rather circular way integrating macro- and microelements. In this section a three-step methodology for understanding the source text is proposed that can be used as a starting point and adapted to your personal style and to the particular needs of each assignment:

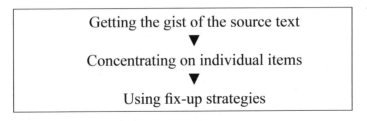

Figure 3.1. A three-step methodology for understanding the source text

Getting the gist of the text

Understanding the main ideas of the source text will enable us to have a comprehensive framework in which to process microelements. However, when trying to get the gist of the text, we may need to understand an individual item – term, expression or sentence. Thus the following strategies can be combined with those presented in the subsection headed 'Concentrating on individual items'.

Using different reading speeds

As professional translators, and readers, we read a variety of documents – source texts, parallel text, dictionaries, books, encyclopaedias, web pages, target texts – and for a variety of purposes – understanding, finding information, revising, and so forth. Therefore, we need to be aware of different types of reading such as scanning, skimming, light-reading, word-by-word reading, study reading, and use them as required (for further information, see Konstant, 2000, and Fink, 2002).

When processing the source text, reading speed should not be uniform. Not all the information contained in the source text is equally relevant. Some items of information are central to the topic of the text, whereas others may be of marginal interest or of lesser importance.

Similarly, you may be familiar with some items of information whereas others may be absolutely new to you. The latter will need to be read more attentively than the former. In other words, allocate more time to what is vital and/or unfamiliar and skip over what is peripheral and/or already known to you.

Outlining and summarizing

Outlining and summarizing can be useful tools to reinforce understanding of the source text. An outline is a sketch giving the prominent features of the source text. It can consist of a linear set of words, expressions or sentences, often loosely linked by lines and arrows, which don't necessarily form a cohesive text. A summary is a cohesive text resulting from the intentional reduction of the content of text from which it is derived. In summaries the most relevant information is kept, and the less relevant information is left out. Thus, one of the key tasks when writing summaries is to identify the main concepts and link them properly with other relevant concepts in the new text. A summary is normally written in the target language and does not necessarily follow the same structure and sequence as that of the original. We can summarize texts in various degrees of quantity and detail: for example, 1/4, 1/2 or 3/4 of the original. When summarizing we should avoid repeating sentences taken literally from the source text. Summarizing often involves paraphrasing and reconnecting information.

Task 11. Outlining and summarizing the source text

1) Look at this example of a summary:

Scientists have developed a new vaccine to treat Alzheimer's disease. They think that the protein beta-amyloid is ultimately responsible for the disease. The vaccine they have devised makes the immune system attack this protein and has no adverse effects in mice.

2) Read the following text:

Renewed Hopes for Vaccine to Treat Alzheimer's

In 2003 preliminary clinical trials of a vaccine to treat Alzheimer's disease were halted because 18 of the 298 patients developed swelling in their brains. The doctors had hoped that by exposing the human immune system to small amounts of beta-amyloid--a protein thought to initiate the buildup of plaques in the brain that underlies the neurodegenerative disease--it could be trained to expel the rogue protein. Instead, in 6 percent of the patients, the immune system overreacted and damaged the brain itself. Now scientists have developed a new DNA-based vaccine that causes cells to produce extra beta-amyloid, thereby engaging the immune system to attack the protein. Plus, when administered to mice, it had no adverse effects. Yoh Matsumoto of the Tokyo Metropolitan Institute for Neuroscience and his colleagues developed the vaccine by tinkering with the DNA that governs beta-amyloid production. The researchers then tested the vaccine *109 Vicent Montalt, María González Davies* under two conditions: as a preventative against development of

plaques and as a therapy once plaques had developed. This meant vac
cinating specially bred mice from the age of three months- before they
had developed plaques--and after 12 months--once plaque cluttering
had begun. After just four months of biweekly injections, mice in the
preventative group had as much as 30 percent less beta-amyloid buildup
than untreated controls had; after a year, up to 50 percent less. "The final
reduction rate of beta amyloid burden in the cerebral cortex at 18 months
of age was roughly 38.5 percent of untreated groups," the team writes
in their report, published online this week by the Proceedings of the
National Academy of Sciences. The DNA vaccine was also effective as
a therapy. After just six months of treatment, it cut beta-amyloid levels
by as much as 40 percent. Most importantly, no matter how often the
vaccine was administered, no brain swelling was observed. "Nonviral
beta-amyloid DNA vaccines are highly effective and safe in reducing
the beta-amyloid burden in model mice and, thus, are promising as a
vaccine therapy against human Alzheimer's disease," the researchers
conclude. --David Biello

(Source: http://www.sciam.com/article.cfm?articleID=000D1595- C153-
148D-80D483414B7F4945)

3) Identify the main concepts and jot them down in the form of an
outline.

4) Write a non-linear summary of the text that takes approximately 1/3
of it.

Text mapping

When processing highly complex contents, text mapping can be an efficient way
of understanding the main concepts and the semantic relationships between them.
A text map is a diagram or symbolic representation of our response to the source
text. Its purpose is to give us a non-linear, hierarchical overview of the content
of the source text. To make a text map, follow these steps:

1. Read the text and underline the main concepts of the topic presented in it.
2. Decide which of them are central and which are peripheral, and list them in
    order of relevance.
3. Write the key concept in the centre of the page.
4. Following the order of relevance write the rest of the concepts around the
    central one.
5. Use lines, arrows and other symbols to represent the main relationships among

them such as cause-effect, time, and space. (When necessary, go back to the source text for information.)

6. Add any details that can help you integrate as much information as possible into the text map.
7. Read the text map aloud in your target language connecting all the elements in it and trying to make sense of the whole.

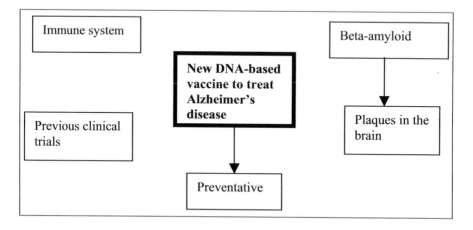

Figure 3.2. Example of text mapping in progress

Task 12. Drawing and using text maps

In the example of text map above (figure 3.2), based on the text in Task 11, there are some important concepts missing. Complete it following the seven instructions given in this subsection.

Exploring metaphors

We use metaphors all the time. We need them both to conceptualize and understand reality and to communicate it to others in a more efficient way. Metaphor, according to Lakoff and Johnson (1980: 115):

> pervades our normal conceptual system. Because so many of the concepts that are important to us are either abstract or nor clearly delineated in our experience [...], we need to get a grasp of them by means of other concepts that we understand in clearer terms.

Metaphors are useful devices for explaining and focusing on specific aspects of complex objects and processes, as can be seen in the following examples:

- The cell is a factory of life and the mitochondrion is seen as the energy plant. In order to prevent attack by external factors, the cell has quality control mechanisms.
- Tumour cells are human beings whose growth and reproduction are abnormal.
- Disease is war and the immune system fights agasinst disease agents.
- Tumour cells invade and colonize different parts of the body.
- The genome is a text. Genetic information is transcribed and translated.

Thus metaphors can be thought of as translations from a source domain of literal, everyday experience into a target domain, with the aim of enlarging and enhancing understanding of that target domain, which is of a more abstract nature (Brown, 2003: 29). Thus in the first example above, an object that we cannot see immediately such as 'cell' (and its parts and functions) is translated into a concept such as 'factory' (and its parts and functions), which we are familiar with in our daily experiences. Metaphors allow us to construct narrative frames from which we can anticipate and infer further elements that come into play. In the first paragraph of the text about a vaccine to treat Alzheimer's (Task 11 above) we can see in the words in bold type how metaphors are used to make us understand the concepts.

> In 2003 preliminary clinical trials of a vaccine to treat Alzheimer's disease were halted because 18 of the 298 patients developed swelling in their brains. The doctors had hoped that by exposing the human immune system to small amounts of beta-amyloid--a protein thought to initiate the buildup of plaques in the brain that underlies the neurodegenerative disease--it could be **trained to expel** the **rogue** protein. Instead, in 6 percent of the patients, the immune system **overreacted** and damaged the brain itself. Now scientists have developed a new DNA-based vaccine that causes cells to produce extra beta-amyloid, thereby engaging the immune system **to attack** the protein. Plus, when administered to mice, it had no adverse effects.

A certain destructive, anomalous and unpredictable protein – 'rogue protein' – attacks the brain. This attack causes a disease, Alzheimer's disease. The researchers try to train the immune system to counter-attack or expel the effect of the rogue protein. Alzheimer's disease is seen, then, as a war between the protein that causes it and the immune system, which in this case is helped by a vaccine. This metaphor-laden style of writing can help us to understand abstract topics more easily. We should also be aware that some metaphors may be politically or socially loaded (see 5.4 *Translating metaphors*).

Concentrating on individual items

Using etymological information

Greek and Latin etymology constitutes a very productive system not only for forming medical terms in many languages, but also for understanding them. Studying and memorizing the most frequent Greek and Latin etymologies of medical roots, suffixes and prefixes (see appendix 2) can be of great help since they are widely used in medical texts. For example, knowing that the prefix 'hypo-' means 'under, below, deficient', and that 'dermis' means 'skin', when you see the expression 'hypodermic injection' in a text you will have enough understanding of it as to integrate it in your mental representation of the text and relate that expression to other semantic elements in the text. Likewise knowing that the suffix '-ectomy' means excision, regardless of the root it combines with you will be able to relate it to a surgical procedure in which a part of the body is cut out, as in 'appendectomy'. Etymological knowledge enables us to infer the key features of medical terms, if not to grasp their meaning fully straight away.

Making inferences and paraphrasing implicit meaning

The source text is the tip of the iceberg. A great deal of information is out of sight and has to be inferred from the surface elements, the surrounding text, the context and the background information in the mind of the reader. In complex texts paraphrasing the implicit meaning can help the reader to understand the content. In this subsection we will look at nominalizations, passive sentences, anaphoric relations, and links between sentences.

• Turning nominalizations into full sentences

Let's look at the following two sentences. They are titles of research articles and as such they try to transmit as much information as possible. The underlined parts of the original titles in 1a and 2a have been paraphrased and expanded in verbal form in 1b and 2b:

1a) <u>Loss of nutrient supply can lead to cell death</u>, loss of matrix production, and increase in matrix degradation and hence to disc degeneration.

1b) Nutrient supplies decrease as a consequence of several causes. This loss of nutrient supply makes some cells die. It also makes…

2a) <u>Excessive growth after epiphyseal plate closure caused by over-secretion of</u>

growth hormone (somatotrophin) results in enlarged hands and feet and an enlarged skull and mandible along with soft tissue enlargement and a number of other endocrine problems.

2b) When growth hormone (somatotrophin) is secreted in excess, epiphyseal plate closure grows excessively. This excessive growth makes...

The result of the paraphrased versions is that the same is said in less abstract, more common sense syntax. Whenever you come across complex nominalizations, try to paraphrase them in verbal form in your target language, so that abstract constructions are turned into common sense expressions which are easier to understand. To paraphrase nominalizations in verbal form you will need to infer some implicit elements (such as the agent of the action expressed by the verb) and state them explicitly, as shown in the examples above.

Task 14. Turning nominalizations into verbal forms

Paraphrase the underlined nominalizations in the following sentences in verbal forms as shown in the examples above.

- Gland removal and hormone replacement stops Graves' disease and other hyperthyroidism.

- The intense sympathetic activation accompanying heart failure stimulates the release of renin from the juxtaglomerular apparatus near the descending loop of Henle in the kidney.

- A reduction in the number of lymphocytes may not cause a significant decrease in the total number of white blood cells.

- Under-secretion of anterior pituitary hormones may cause Simmonds' disease and dwarfism.

- Turning passive sentences into active sentences

In passive sentences the subject of the verb has been deleted and the reader's job is made a little harder. Inferring the subject and making it explicit can help us to understand a text quicker: Consider the following examples:

1a) However, in most cases, other methods are employed to insure reduction of hyperglycaemia.

1b) However, in most cases, doctors employ other methods to insure reduction of hyperglycaemia.

2a) [The adrenal medulla receives messages from the brain through a nerve. In response to stimulation along nerves of the sympathetic nervous system the adrenal medulla releases the catecholamines epinephrine (adrenaline) and norepinephrine (noradrenaline).] These hormones <u>are released</u> in stressful situations as part of the 'flight / fight' mechanism.

2b) <u>The adrenal medulla</u> <u>releases</u> these hormones in stressful situations as part of the 'flight / fight' mechanism.

• Exploring anaphoric relations and making word substitutions

We all know that pronouns can replace nouns and refer neatly back to something already mentioned. But sometimes synonyms or phrases can function in a similar way. In the first example, 'this ischaemia' refers back to 'reduces the blood supply to the legs', and 'these affected parts' refers back to 'feet or lower leg':

> Atherosclerosis of the abdominal aorta, the iliac, and the femoral arteries invariably reduces the blood supply to the legs (1). As a consequence of this ischemia (1), diabetic patients often experience cold feet and legs as well as ulcers of the feet and lower legs. Eventually, the reduced blood flow may lead to gangrene of the feet or lower leg (2). Amputation of these affected parts (2) is too often the unfortunate outcome of diabetes mellitus.

In the second example, 'the same concentration' refers back to '0.1mM or ~19.3 mg/l MDMA':

> The lowest concentration that impaired cell functioning in these studies (0.1mM or ~19.3 mg/l MDMA) affected indices of cell viability after 24, but not 6, hours in the study by Beitia et al (2000). The same concentration had no significant pro-fibrogenic effect after 24 hr in the study by Varela-Rey et al (1999).

This referring back is called anaphoric deixis, and is very common in medical texts. Substituting these anaphoric elements with the words or expressions they refer to can help to enhance understanding in complex texts.

Task 15. Identifying anaphoric elements

Identify and paraphrase the underlined anaphors in the following sentences:

• Hyperadrenalism (Cushing's Syndrome) is a condition caused by

---

hypersecretion of adrenal cortex hormones. Cushing's patients have the triad of moon face, buffalo hump, and striae. In addition, they have prolonged wound repair. It is caused by over-secretion of ACTH or by prolonged use of corticosteroid medications to control some serious condition (e.g. pemphigus vulgaris). Removal of these hormones will stop Cushing's syndrome.

- Patients with hypoadrenalism from whatever cause show pigmentation, weakness, hypotension, loss of appetite, and loss of weight. If these features are particularly prominent, the term "Addison's disease" is applied.
- When you have diabetes, your body either doesn't make enough insulin or can't use its own insulin as well as it should, or both. This causes sugars to build up too high in your blood.
- As the ventricles contract, the blood is forced in a retrograde fashion against the AV valves, which causes them to bulge inward slightly toward the atria and which also elevates atrial pressure. In doing so, the AV valves are effectively closed and blood is prevented from regurgitating back into the atria.

- Exploring links between and within sentences

Sentences can be linked with one another and within themselves in different ways. Cause-effect relationships are very common, as in the following examples:

> *Helicobacter pylori* (*H. pylori*) infection is acquired in childhood, earlier in developing countries; as a consequence the prevalence of infection is higher in developing countries (70%) than in developed countries (5-15%).

> People with diabetes have an abnormal elevation of their blood sugar, and lack adequate insulin to metabolize the blood sugar. As a consequence, the blood glucose (sugar) abnormally enters certain nerve tissue and damages the nerve.

We must ensure that we identify the cause and the effect, and relate them by means of the linking word. The links between and within sentences can also express other semantic relationships: addition; opposition, antithesis or difference; position in time or space; or a combination of them. These links are useful signals which help us we connect the main semantic elements of the sentence appropriately.

Sometimes the connection between sentences or parts of the same sentence is not made explicit and we need to look for the link in the surrounding text.

> There is <u>more than one</u> disease known by the term "diabetes." "<u>Diabetes insipidus</u>" is an uncommon disease caused by undersecretion of antidiuretic hormone (ADH) and characterized by increased urine production (diabetes) unaccompanied by elevations in blood and urine sugar. <u>Diabetes mellitus</u>, **on the other hand**, is such a common disorder that when the term "diabetes" is used, diabetes mellitus is meant.

In this particular example there is a gap between the first and the second sentences in which the following linking expression can be inferred: 'There is more than one disease known by the term "diabetes." On the one hand, "Diabetes insipidus" is...'

Chunking long sentences

Dividing long sentences into shorter ones is a very useful strategy which breaks down complex information into more manageable chunks and therefore helps us to understand the source text more easily. To form new sentences from the original one we usually need to make explicit both conceptual and syntactic or connective information. This strategy may require some of the other strategies presented above, such as turning nominalizations into full sentences, identifying deixis, or exploring links.

Example:

> Reduction in nephron mass from the initial injury reduces the glomerular filtration rate (GFR), leading to hypertrophy and hyperfiltration of the remaining nephrons and to the initiation of intraglomerular hypertension in order to increase the GFR of the remaining nephrons, thus minimizing the functional consequences of nephron loss.
> When kidneys are injured, nephron mass is reduced. This reduction in nephron mass leads to hypertrophy and hyperfiltration of the remaining nephrons and to the initiation of intraglomerular hypertension. These changes occur in order to increase the GFR of the remaining nephrons. This increase minimizes the functional consequences of nephron loss.

This comprehension strategy may sometimes lead to a translation procedure which consists of turning one long sentence in the source text into several shorter sentences in the target text (see section 4.4 Crafting your target text).

Activating one particular sense of a polysemic term

Medical terms can be polysemic. Context and surrounding text enable us to decide which sense of a particular term is activated in a particular instance.

Task 16. Understanding polysemic terms

1) Look at the following definitions of 'drug' in the *Dorlands Medical Dictionary*:

1. a chemical substance that affects the processes of the mind or body.
2. any chemical compound used on or administered to humans or animals as an aid in the diagnosis, treatment, or prevention of disease or other abnormal condition, for the relief of pain or suffering, or to control or improve any physiologic or pathologic condition.
3. a substance used recreationally for its effects on the central nervous system, such as a narcotic; abuse may lead to dependence or addiction.

2) Which one of them is activated in the following text? Explain why.

On April 7, 2005, the Food and Drug Administration (FDA) announced that they are asking manufacturers of all prescription nonsteroidal anti-inflam-matory **drugs** (NSAIDs) to revise the **drug** labeling (package insert) to include a ''boxed'' or serious warning about the potential for increased risk of cardiovascular events (including heart attack and stroke) and serious and potentially life-threatening gastrointestinal (GI) bleeding associated with their use. This information will also state that patients who have just had heart surgery should not take these medications. The FDA is also asking manu-facturers of nonprescription (OTC) NSAIDs to include information on the product label about the potential for cardiovascular events and GI bleeding, as well as skin reactions in patients taking these **drugs**. You should talk to your doctor if you are taking one of these **drugs** and have any questions or concerns about this new information. For more information visit the FDA website: http://www.fda.gov/cder/drug/infopage/COX2/default.htm.

Fix-up strategies

Monitoring our own understanding is a vital part of reading comprehension. But what can we do if we still can't understand the text? Once we recognize that we are stuck, we can use the following strategies identified by Herrell and Jordan (2002: 226) to help us to clarify the meaning of the text:

- Ignoring the problem and continuing to read, hoping that something in the following text will clarify the text that's not understood.
- Suspending judgement for now and continuing to read with the idea that connections will be made clear at a later point in the text (slightly different from the previous approach in that it's the connections between or among

elements in the story that are not making sense rather than a particular sentence or phrase).

- Forming a tentative hypothesis based on information in the text and then continuing to read to confirm or revise your hypothesis.
- Looking back or rereading the previous sentence.
- Stopping and thinking about the meaning of the previously read material and rereading it in an attempt to fit it into the bigger picture.
- Seeking help from resources such as dictionaries, reference materials, and knowledgeable people. This set of strategies is addressed in chapter 6. In the rest of this section we will simply introduce one of the commonest fix-up strategies.

Consulting definitions of terms in monolingual dictionaries and encyclopaedias

A definition is a precise statement that summarizes the main elements of the meaning of a concept. Definitions are extremely useful for medical translators, especially when we are not familiar with the topic of the text. They may range from very basic ones addressed to the general public, to highly specialized ones addressed to experts in the field. Here we have three different definitions of 'synapse' from different terminological sources meant for different purposes and readers:

1) 'The point at which a nervous impulse passes from one neuron to another.'
   (Source: *Merriam Webster OnLine* <http://www.m-w.com>)

2) 'The point of connection usually between two nerve cells. Specifically, a synapse is a specialized junction at which a nerve cell (a neuron) communicates with a target cell. The neuron releases a chemical transmitter (a neurotransmitter) that diffuses across a small gap and activates specific specialized sites called receptors situated on the target cell. The target cell may be another neuron, or a specialized region of a muscle cell or a secretory cell (a cell than can make and secrete a substance). Neurons can also communicate through direct electrical connections (electrical synapses).'
   (Source: *MedicineNet.com* <http://www.medicinenet.com>)

3) 'The site of functional apposition between neurons, at which an impulse is transmitted from one neuron to another, usually by a chemical neurotransmitter (e.g., acetylcholine, norepinephrine, etc.) released by the axon terminal of the excited (presynaptic) cell. The neurotransmitter diffuses across the synaptic cleft to bind with receptors on the postsynaptic cell membrane, and thereby effects electrical changes in the postsynaptic cell which result in depolarization (excitation) or hyperpolarization (inhibition). Synapses also

occur at sites of apposition between nerve endings and effector organs (e.g., the neuromuscular junction). A few synapses in the central nervous system are electrical synapses (q.v.). In official terminology called synapsis.

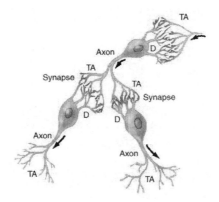

Diagram of three synapses. Nerve impulse is indicated by arrows, show-ing that the direction of passage is from the terminal arborization (TA) or nerve endings of the axon of one neuron to the dendrites (D) of another neuron.
(Source, Dorland's Medical Dictionary at <http://www.merksource. com>)

In the rest of the definition different types of synapses – such as 'axoaxonic', 'axodentritic', 'electrotonic', and so forth – are presented and explained. When processing the source text we may just need brief information of a particular term which is not of central importance in the whole text. When we are dealing with key terms – terms that are constantly referred to and expanded along the text – then we may need longer, more detailed definitions.

3.4 Further tasks

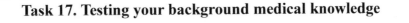

Task 17. Testing your background medical knowledge

This task is designed to help you become aware of your knowledge and experience in the medical field and it can be used as a diagnos-tic tool at an initial stage. Choose at least two of the following and define them in your target language. If necessary, use a knowledge resource (see chapter 6) to find basic information about them.
- Laboratory tests
- Allergic and immunological disorders
- Blood diseases

- Cardiovascular disorders
- Cavity and membrane disorders
- Congenital and hereditary diseases
- Connective tissue disorders
- Ear and hearing disorders
- Endocrine disorders
- Excretory system disorders
- Eye and vision disorders
- Gastrointestinal disorders
- Hepatic and biliary disorders
- Infectious diseases caused by bacteria and related organisms
- Infectious diseases caused by fungi
- Infectious diseases caused by parasites
- Infectious diseases caused by viruses
- Lymphatic system disorders
- Muscle disorders
- Nervous system disorders
- Nutritional diseases
- Oral disorders
- Pregnancy related disorders
- Reproductive disorders
- Respiratory system disorders
- Sexually transmitted diseases
- Skeletal disorders
- Skin disorders

3.5 Further reading

Brown, Gillian, Kirsten Malmkjær, Alastair Pollitt and John Williams (eds) (1994) *Language and Understanding* Oxford: Oxford University Press.

Brown, Theodore L. (2003) *Making Truth: Metaphor in Science*, Urbana and Chicago: University of Illinois Press.

Gylys, Barbara A. and Mary Ellen Wedding (2005) *Medical Terminology Systems. A Body Systems Approach*, Philadelphia: F.A. Davies Company, 5th edition.

Herrell, Adrienne and Michael Jordan (2002) *Active Learning Strategies for Improving Reading Comprehension*, New Jersey and Ohio: Merrill Prentice Hall.

Jackendoff, R (1983) *Semantics and Cognition*, Cambridge and London: Massachusetts Institute of Technology.

Kintsch, Walter (1998) *Comprehension. A Paradigm for Cognition*, Cambridge: Cambridge University Press.

Konstant, Tina (2000) *Speed Reading*, London: Hodder Headline.

Lakoff, George and Mark Johnson (1980) *Metaphors We Live By*, Chicago: University of Chicago Press.

------ (1999) *Philosophy in the Flesh: The Embodied Mind and its Challenge to Western Thought*, New York: Basic Books.

Sontag, Susan (1991) *Illness as Metaphor. Aids and its Metaphors*, London: Penguin.

Van Rijn-van Tongeren, G.W. (1997) *Metaphors in Medical Texts*, Amsterdam: Rodopi. [Utrecht Studies in Language and Communication]

Further reading by body systems

General

<http://health.nhi.gov>
<http://www.medicalstudent.com>

Integumentary system

<http://www.cancerindex.org/medterm/medtm5.htm#function>
<http://www.zoology.ubc.ca/~biomania/tutorial/skin/outline.htm>
<http://www.nlm.nih.gov/medlineplus/skinhairandnails.html>
<http://www.merck.com/mrkshared/mmanual/section10/sec10.jsp>

Digestive system

<http://www.innerbody.com/image/digeov.html>
<http://www.nlm.nih.gov/medlineplus/digestivesystem.html>
<http://www.nlm.nih.gov/medlineplus/mouthandteeth.html>
<http://www.merck.com/mrkshared/mmanual/section3/sec3.jsp>
<http://www.merck.com/mrkshared/mmanual/section4/sec4.jsp>

Respiratory system

<http://www.le.ac.uk/pa/teach/va/anatomy/frmst.html>
<http://www.nlm.nih.gov/medlineplus/lungsandbreathing.html>
<http://www.merck.com/mrkshared/mmanual/section6/sec6.jsp>

Cardiovascular system

<http://www.innerbody.com/image/cardov.html>
<http://cardiovascular.cx>
<http://www.merck.com/mrkshared/mmanual/section16/sec16.jsp>
<http://www.nlm.nih.gov/medlineplus/ency/article/000147.htm>

<http://health.nhi.gov>
<http://www.medicalstudent.com>

Blood, lymph, and immune systems

<http://www.thebody.com/nih/immune_system.html>
<http://www.nlm.nih.gov/medlineplus/immunesystemanddisorders.html>
<http://www.nlm.nih.gov/medlineplus/immunesystem.html>
<http://www.nlm.nih.gov/medlineplus/ency/article/002247.htm>
<http://www.lymphnotes.com/article.php/id/151>
<http://kidshealth.org/parent/general/body_basics/blood.html>
<http://www.nlm.nih.gov/medlineplus/bloodandblooddisorders.html>

Female reproductive system

<http://www.emc.maricopa.edu/faculty/farabee/BIOBK/BioBookREPROD.
    html>
<http://training.seer.cancer.gov/module_anatomy/unit12_3_repdt_female.
    html>
<http://www.nlm.nih.gov/medlineplus/femalereproductivesystem.html>
<http://www.merck.com/mmhe/sec22/ch241/ch241a.html>

Endocrine system

<http://www.vivo.colostate.edu/hbooks/pathphys/endocrine/index.html>
<http://www.innerbody.com/image/endoov.html>
<http://www.emc.maricopa.edu/faculty/farabee/biobk/BioBookENDOCR.html>
<http://www.nlm.nih.gov/medlineplus/endocrinesystem.html>

Nervous system

<http://www.nlm.nih.gov/medlineplus/brainandnerves.html>
<http://www.getbodysmart.com/ap/nervoussystem/nervoussystem.html>
<http://www-edu.net>
<http://www.ama-assn.org/ama/pub/category/7172.html>

4. Drafting the target text

> You will need more than one draft; all writers who want to write accurately and clearly revise again and again.
>
> Edward J. Huth (1999: 121)

Overview of chapter

When we draft the target text, we are making a rough sketch from which the final copy is made; that is, a delineation of a text – giving the prominent features of its structure and contents without full detail – which is intended to serve as the basis of a finished text. But before starting to write the draft (4.1), we will briefly look at the general principles that should guide the overall process. It may also be useful to become aware of our own writing styles and to become familiar with some of the methods used by successful medical writers. Only when we have defined the assignment and have an adequate understanding of the source text, can we start drafting the target text. A three-step drafting methodology (4.2) – composing, crafting and improving – that takes into account the target genre's restrictions and possibilities, can be applied to any medical genre. The first step, composing the target text (4.3), focuses on the overall structure and content. Once structure and content are in the first draft, we can then move on to crafting specific aspects of the target text (4.4) such as paragraphing, cohesive devices, modality, phraseology and titling conventions. The next step will be improving the draft (4.5) paying special attention to semantic, pragmatic and stylistic aspects that may affect the readability and acceptability of the target text. Both genre shift in the process of translation (4.6), also referred to in the literature as heterofunctional or transgeneric translation, and the translation of research papers into English (4.7) deserve special attention owing to their growing relevance in professional practice. Some tasks (4.8) and suggestions for further reading (4.9) are presented at the end of the chapter.

4.1 Before starting to write

General principles

In the process of drafting the target text we have to take many decisions. The following principles are intended as a guide. No matter what the specifics of the assignment are, the target text should be:

- Coherent with the source text as far as factual information is concerned

- Coherent internally so that the information hangs together in a logical order
- Truthful and accurate – corresponding with fact or reality
- Readable, so that the reader can process the information without undue effort
- Clear – as easy to understand as possible
- Grammatically and syntactically correct
- Adequate – stylistically and rhetorically in keeping with the communicative situation and context.

Styles of drafting: Are you a hare or a tortoise?

Before beginning to draft the target text, we have to weigh up the advantages and disadvantages of starting to write before dealing with some or all of the comprehension gaps. Our deliberations will be influenced by three factors: our perception of the degree of difficulty of the source text; our degree of familiarity with the topic and terminology; and the complexity of the assignment in terms of formal and communicative differences between the source and the target texts.

Starting to write the draft before fully understanding the source text:	*Starting to write the draft only after fully understanding the source text:*
Advantages	*Advantages*
Although our draft will probably have many gaps, at least we have something from which to start researching and improving.	We will probably feel more secure and empowered to write a target text which makes sense to our reader. We will also be able to write with fewer interruptions.
Disadvantages	*Disadvantages*
Without understanding the key concepts, it is impossible to follow the narrations, descriptions or arguments of the source text and connect them into a relevant whole. Therefore it becomes difficult to link microelements and make inferences. We may also feel insecure when writing the target text and may tend to produce literal translations when lost.	The information acquired and the solutions found to specific problems during documentary research need to be retained in note form or in the memory. This takes time and effort.

Figure 4.1. When to start drafting the target text

Of course, there is not only one method of drafting and, like other writers, translators have their own individual preferences. Nevertheless, writers seem to fall into two main types as far as writing the target text is concerned: hares and tortoises.

Hares are impatient. They want to be off in this race against time. They don't want to stop to think carefully. Getting to the end is all-important. So they write down everything they can as quickly as possible. But their initial drafts are pretty dreadful. All the same, they are reassured because they feel they've made a start.

Tortoises take their time but get there in the end. They approach things carefully and they spent a great deal of time thinking about what they're writing, which means that they aim at something approaching a finished text. They revise constantly as they go along. They make slow progress but the first draft is robust and largely error-free.

These two extreme cases are rather unrealistic stereotypes and few writers are exclusively one or the other. Different genres and different assignments may lend themselves better to one approach than the other or even to a combination of both. For example, a genre shift (see 4.6 Genre shift) may require a slower approach with repeated revisions until all elements of structure and language are satisfactorily adjusted, whereas translating a familiar, highly conventionalized genre may require a faster, more linear approach in which very little is left for further revision.

Another factor in the choice of approach may be experience, or the lack of it. Experienced translators may prefer to write a fairly polished first draft which needs minor editing and revision, whereas inexperienced translators and students may feel more comfortable and confident working step by step through a number of drafts. The methodology that we present in this chapter is addressed to the latter.

Task 1. What's your writing style?

In your next translation assignment, try to become aware of your working style using the information in this subsection. Then decide in which ways your working style could be rebalanced between the two extremes described above in order to improve your performance as a medical translator.

What successful writers in the biomedical fields do

Medical translation is, of course, a type of medical writing. According to the literature on medical writing, professionals do not write at random but use techniques such as:

- Listing topics dealt with in the text
- Drawing concept maps (clustering, branching)
- Drawing issue trees
- Outlining
- Drafting (following standard structure)
- Starting in the place that makes sense for them
- Minimizing distractions any way they can
- Keeping the text simple
- When really pressed, spending more time on the first draft, not less
- Writing around missing information
- Recognizing the signs of becoming bogged down
- Dealing constructively with writer's block.

Medical translators can definitely benefit from these and other techniques used by medical writers. As we can see from the list above, professional writers don't necessarily start at the beginning and plod through to the end, but they work methodically nevertheless. Without a methodology for drafting the target text, translators – particularly inexperienced ones – may be less aware of what they're doing and run the risk of focusing too much on microelements, both of which may result in literal and useless renderings of the source text. Hence the importance of developing a methodology in which the source text is viewed just as factual information – 'offer of information' in Nord's terminology – and the target text is produced with intended meaning and function regarded as of paramount importance.

4.2 A drafting methodology

In order to perform a piece of music properly, musicians rehearse the score, dissecting it, paying attention to particular aspects (rhythm, phrasing, sound quality, etc.), and then integrate everything back into a complex, meaningful whole, which is what we hear in the performance. Likewise, in medical writing, attention is paid to specific aspects of the text production process – readership analysis, organization of content, formal structure, first draft, in-house style norms, revision, and so forth – before everything is integrated into the finished product.

In medical translation practice and training, the focus has traditionally been on the result of the process, and more particularly on terminology, rather than on exploring the different operations that take place in the course of writing of the target text. Many of these operations are complex, difficult to describe and often take place simultaneously. But we need to look at them separately if we are to learn more about them in practical terms. By paying attention to the various parts of the writing process we can gain insights and improve our performance.

Sometimes problems arise and remain to be dealt with – or in the worst cases, are left unresolved – in the finished text. But many such difficulties could be avoided by following a positive and effective drafting methodology which can nip problems in the bud. The information and experience offered here should be taken as a starting point, a sound foundation, but not as prescription of what all medical translators should do.

We will approach the draft positively concentrating on the possibilities available to us rather than analyzing the finished text in negative terms (as problems). The draft is the skeleton which we will later flesh out and clothe as appropriate.

We should avoid trying to produce a polished text at the first attempt, as if good writing were a linear, irreversible process focused only on microelements. It is not. It would be better to make a series of sketches of growing factual and formal detail, which will eventually result in the finished target text. Drafting and re-drafting is a positive and useful aid to improving and refining a text, and if it is done systematically, it can cut down on the time spent on later revisions. In addition, drafting enables us to have a broader and richer view of overall information structure and progression. Finally this drafting methodology can open professional opportunities – for example, increased expertise in editing original texts.

Drafting in three steps: composing, crafting and improving

Hedge (2005) establishes a number of tasks that writers perform during the process of *original writing*:

Being motivated to write	>	Getting ideas together	>	Planning and outlining	>	Making notes	>	Making a first draft	>	Revising Replanning Redrafting	>	Editing and getting ready for publication

Figure 4.2. The writing process (Hedge, 2005: 51)

As far as drafting is concerned, however, *translating* is a particular type of writing that differs only in some minor details from the above process:

Assignment	>	Understanding the source text	>	Planning and outlining	>	Making a first draft	>	Revising Replanning Redrafting	>	Editing and getting ready for publication

Figure 4.3. The translation process

As we can see, except for the first two activities, the rest are exactly the same. Aspects relating to the assignment and the comprehension of the source text have been dealt with in chapters 1 and 3 respectively. In this chapter we examine the rest of the steps just as they could be approached in any other writing process, that is, moving gradually from general aspects of structure and content to more specific details of grammar and style. Let us then consider a drafting methodology based on the following three steps:

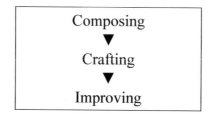

Figure 4.4. A three-step drafting methodology

Although here these three steps are presented one after the other, in real practice they often overlap and feed back to one another in a circular way.

We have chosen this methodology (following Hedge, 2005) because it allows us to focus on different elements of the process in a systematic way and because it embraces full translation as is traditionally understood as well as other writing tasks – from editing and adapting the source text, to genre shifts, to original writing – that medical translators need to master to meet the demands of the market.

4.3 Composing your target text

It is often assumed that the way a text is organized and structured depends only on the source-text author and that a translator should not meddle with it in any way.

However, working through the target text in an exclusively linear, bottom-up way – word after word, sentence after sentence, paragraph after paragraph – and assuming that structure has nothing to do with the translator, may not be the best strategy. There are two main reasons for this: 1) changes of structure may be needed in the assignment; 2) even if structural changes are not a real need, working top-down – from structure to word choice – may be a more effective and insightful approach.

In the first place, macro and micro structural adjustments are often needed: the conventional structure of the target genre may be different from that of the source genre; we may have to change the paragraph divisions; we may have to alter the internal order of a paragraph or even the order of paragraphs. The reasons may be poor writing in the source text or simply different rhetorical conventions in the target language (as pointed out by Mossop, 2001: 61), and also the demands of particular assignments in which genre shifts are involved (see section 4.6).

Secondly, more often than is commonly thought, solutions to particular problems may be in a different place within the text. For example, explanations of complex concepts, networks of concepts, cause and effect relationships, argumentations, repetition of particular collocations, and terminological preferences can only be discovered if we develop an overall view of text progression.

Thus, instead of translating from beginning to end in a linear way, we could start by composing the overall structure of the target text, that is, the sum of the parts that make up the whole. Sometimes those parts are physically indicated by means of section and subsection headings. In those cases we are lucky because we have a ready-made template that is very useful for our writing purposes. Sometimes those parts are not overtly signalled, which means that we have to discover the structural pattern for ourselves. Recognizing structural patterns or templates whether they are explicit or not, and using them in the drafting process is the main purpose of this section.

When we compose the target text we organize different types of information into a template, which works as a pattern or gauge that we use as a starting point and a guide when drafting the target text. These templates are to a greater or lesser degree standardized and conventionalized. That is, their different parts, the types of information they contain, the functions they fulfil, and the terminology and phraseology they normally use can be highly predictable. For example, in the "Undesirable effects" section of the summary of product characteristics (see chapter 2), statements such as the following are commonly repeated:

> "Approximately .....% of patients can be expected to experience adverse reactions. These are mainly dose dependent and due to the pharmacological effects of the medicinal product."

> "At the beginning of therapy, epigastric pain, nausea, diarrhoea, headache or vertigo may occur: these reactions are usually mild and disappear within a few days even if treatment is continued."

Becoming familiar with the templates means being able to interiorize them, to anticipate them in the translation process and turn them into habits when drafting the target text, and, as a consequence, gaining confidence as a writer. Seen from this perspective, our target text is an existing template, which we fill with information from the source text to produce a new text.

The information contained in the template can be related in different ways (timewise, spacewise, and so forth.) Being aware of overall information patterns enhances target text cohesion and communicative purpose. In the table below Matthews et al. suggest common patterns for organizing information in medical genres that can help us become aware of text structure:

Pattern	Basis
Chronological	The sequence in which something happened
Geographical or spatial	The physical arrangement of entities
Functional	How parts work
Importance	Usually with elements in order of decreasing importance
Possible solutions	From least to most likely or best, or building to a climax
Specificity	General to particular, or particular to general
Complexity	Usually from simple to complex
Pros and cons	Presenting both sides of an issue or decisions
Causality	Cause and effect

Figure 4.5. Organizational patterns in writing
(Matthews et al, 2000: 57)

It is a good idea to be aware of these patterns so that we can understand how the source text is organized and how to proceed when composing the target text. Composing involves outlining a structure and filling it with the information provided by the source text. But before we move on to outlining standard structures, let's test our immediate sense of structure.

Task 2. Creating structure

Imagine you have just been diagnosed with a particular disease, say Crohn's disease, Parkinson's disease, or any other. What would you want to find out about it? What questions would you ask a physician?

1)   Write them down as they occur to you.

2) Now put them into a logical order.
3) Examine why you think your order is logical. These questions will constitute the structure of your target text.
4) Decide which of the patterns in Figure 4.5 best fits the structure you have created.
5) Look for information in English about the disease you have chosen.
6) Answer the questions you have asked in your target language.
7) Look for a fact sheet about the disease and compare its structure with the one you have created.
8) Decide whether you would alter it in any way after reading the fact sheet.

If you look at other fact sheets you will see that there is a recognizable pattern in them. They are examples of standard structures which can be helpful drafting devices because they provide a clear idea of text progression and overall coherence. Three genres will be explored: fact sheet for patients, summary of product characteristics, and original article. Both summaries of product characteristics and original articles have highly standardized structures, whereas there may be considerable variations in fact sheets for patients and patient information leaflets not only between languages but also within the same language (see chapter 2).

Fact sheets for patients are used to give patients information about their disease or condition and its treatment, among other things. Their typical macrostructure consists of the following sections, each of them containing a different type of information:

- Research: Have researchers come up with any relevant findings for the understanding, treatment or prevention of the disease?
- Treatment: Can it be cured or controlled or alleviated? How? Pharmacological treatment, gene therapy, diet, exercise, psychotherapy, physiotherapy, etc.?
- Complications: What are the effects of the disease? What adverse effect does it have on patients? In which percentages? (statistical information) Does it affect particular population groups (sex, age, ethnic origin, geographical origin, etc.) more than others?
- Overview: What does the disease consist of? What is it exactly? What is it not? Are there different types? Which? How do they differ from each other? What can the outcomes of the disease be?
- Prevalence: How many people suffer from this disease? What is their geographical distribution?
- Diagnosis: How can the disease be detected in patients?
- Risk factors: What other conditions can increase the chances of contracting the disease? And in which order of importance?

- Prevention: Can the onset of the disease be delayed or even avoided? How?
- Causes: Is it inherited? Is it acquired? How? Is there a chain of different causes and effects leading to the disease?
- Signs and symptoms: How does it manifest itself? How visible are the signs and symptoms?

Task 3. Rearranging the order of information in the target text

The above sections have been written down in a random order. But they might have been ordered differently had the readers been taken into consideration.

1) Rearrange them more logically and coherently so that their order makes sense to your target reader.
2) Translate them into your mother tongue.

As mentioned above, these sections, their sequence and the types of information they contain may vary depending both on the subject matter of the fact sheet and on the organization that issues it. Compare the structure in the following fact sheets about diabetes mellitus issued by the *World Health Organization* and by *Patient UK*:

World Health Organization	*Patient UK*
• Diabetes mellitus • Symptoms • Prevalence • Diagnosis • Treatment • Complications associated with diabetes mellitus • Prevention • Related links	• What is diabetes? • Understanding blood glucose and insulin • Type 1 diabetes • Type 2 diabetes • What are the symptoms of Type 2 diabetes? • How is diabetes diagnosed? • What are the possible complications of diabetes • What are the aims of treatment? • Treatment aim 1 – keeping your blood glucose down

	• Treatment aim 2 – to reduce other risk factors • Treatment aim 3 – to detect early and treat any complications • Immunisation • Diabetes UK • Related pages

Figure 4.6. Comparison of two structures of fact sheets for patients

Some other genres show a much more conventionalized structure, which both medical writers and translators must observe. For example, the structure, the types of information contained, and even the headings of the different sections of summaries of product characteristics (see chapter 2) in the European Union are standardized by law (see Article 4a of Directive 65/65/EEC). The summary of product characteristics is one of the genres you are most likely to translate in professional practice, hence the importance of being familiar with its structure (see chapter 2).

Task 4. Writing an outline

1) Go to 'Summary of Product Characteristics (SPC)' in section 5 of chapter 2 and translate into your mother tongue the section and subsection headings contained in figure 2.11.
2) See at <http://www.emea.org> whether your mother tongue is on the list of the languages used by EMEA.
3) If it is, revise your translation taking the official one as the correct one. Every time you translate a summary of product characteristics, you will use this structure and these headings to name its parts.

Now we move down one more level and see how in this example the fourth section of this genre (clinical particulars) unfolds in different subsections also defined by law in full detail:

4.1 Therapeutic indications
4.2 Posology and method of administration
4.3 Contraindications
4.4 Special warnings and special precautions for use
4.5 Interaction with other medicaments and other forms of interaction
4.6 Pregnancy and lactation

4.7 Effects on ability to drive or use machines
4.8 Undesirable effects
4.9 Overdose

Descending one more level we see that, for example, in '4.5 Interaction with other medicaments and other forms of interaction' we might find one of the following three recommendations (see the description of the SPC in chapter 2):

- Contraindication of concomitant use
- Concomitant use not recommended
- Precautions

Let us look now at another genre: the original article. When composing the structure of the target text we must always be guided by the specific communicative purpose and kind of information of each of the parts of the structure. Although the structure of original papers is not determined by law, it is highly conventionalized thanks to the efforts of the editors of biomedical research journals which have an international readership (for further information on this topic, see section 4.7 in this chapter).

1. **Introduction:** the area of knowledge and the particular problem or question addressed. In this section authors tell readers why they have undertaken the study, and what their study adds to previous studies.
2. **Materials and methods:** the experiment and its credibility. In this section authors describe, in logical sequence, how the study was designed and carried out, and how they analyzed the data.
3. **Results:** the evidence itself and the initial answer to the problem or question addressed. Here authors answer the question 'what was found?'.
4. **Discussion:** the meaning of the results. In this section authors examine the evidence for and against, and any supporting evidence from other studies. Finally they assess all evidence and provide an answer to the initial question.

Task 5. Transforming structures in the composing process

1) Go to <http://www.annals.org>, click on 'Past issues', click on a year with free access, and find a 'Summary for patients' of an 'Original article'.
2) Read it carefully, paying special attention to the different sections and the type of information they contain.

3) Go to <http://www.bjm.com> and choose an original article that covers a topic you are interested in.
4) Read it carefully and underline the information that is most relevant for the patients.
5) Compose a text in your target language that has the structure, types of information, and function of the summary for patients you have seen at <http://www.annals.org>.

Organizing types of information and their purpose

We now move on and see how a *specific section* of a genre works, in this case, the *introduction* of original articles. Look at the text below taken from the *British Medical Journal* (vol. 326, May 2003 <http://bmj.com>).

> In many developed countries the number of prescriptions for antidepressants increased steeply during the 1990s, after the introduction of selective serotonin reuptake inhibitors (SSRIs). In some countries, such as Sweden and Hungary, the increased rate of prescribing coincided with a fall in the suicide rate.
> We examined the association between antidepressant prescribing in Australia and changes in rates of suicide for 1991-2000. We analysed differences in suicide trends between men and women in different age groups to assess whether age and sex rates in suicide were related to exposure to antidepressant medication, or to a change in that exposure over time.

The information in the text is structured in the following way:

A) *Type of information and purpose organized logically*	B) *Specific linguistic realization*
1) Review of previous research	'In many developed ... with fall in the suicide rate'
2) Identification of a gap in research which needs to be filled	'We examined the association ... 1991-2000'
3) Objective of the study	'to assess whether ... in that exposure over time'

Figure 4.7. An example of a three-move introduction to an original article

Swales has researched this area of writing and he refers to these logically organized items in column A as 'moves'. Since this terminology is widely used in training manuals for academic writing and has also been taken up by authors in the field of Translation Studies, this term will be the one we shall use in future. Here is a definition of moves provided by Swales (2000: 35):

> *Move* is a functional term that refers to a defined and bounded communicative act that is designed to achieve one main communicative objective. Because it is a functional category the length of a move can range from a single finite clause to several paragraphs.

In other words, one communicative act in a research article may be expressed in a sentence (e.g. the objective of a research paper, which normally takes only one sentence, two at the most), a paragraph (e.g. a brief review of the literature pertaining to the area of the research topic), or indeed, may take even longer to express and need several paragraphs (e.g. a complex argument involving several layers each of which may need its own paragraph but which are still part of the same argument) and therefore these several paragraphs still constitute one move.

In the table above the moves in column A are shared by the languages involved in any scientific translation process. Those in B are specific linguistic realizations of each of the moves. Clearly, realizations will vary both within one language and between languages. It goes without saying that the integrity of the content of the source text must be respected.

The three-move pattern or template illustrated in our example is not an isolated case, but is in fact the norm in introductions of original articles in the biomedical field. In other words, the type of information and communicative purpose are not up to the particular author of this text, but are conventions of the genre shared by many authors. What the author controls are the linguistic realizations reflecting those purposes as well as the new factual information which is transmitted to the target reader.

Furthermore, Swales points out that this pattern is quite regular and stable in most research articles across many disciplines. In the following figure – which may be seen as a more expanded model of what we saw in our specific example in figure 4.1 – we can see how introductions of original articles are internally structured by means of moves.

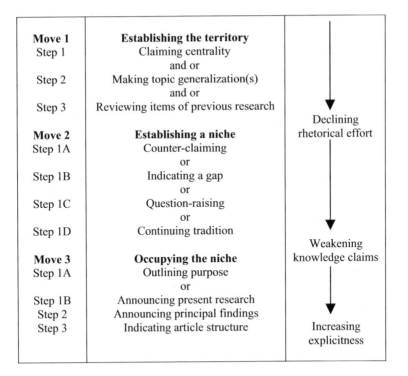

Figure 4.8. Three-move CARS model (Swales, 1990 as cited by Bhatia, 1993)

Just as a genre has a communicative purpose (see chapter 2) in the same way moves also fulfil communicative purposes within particular genres.

Task 6. Identifying and drafting moves in introductions of original articles

1) Choose an original article from any journal you find interesting at <http:// www.freemedicaljournals.com>.
2) Read the introduction carefully. To what extent does it follow the pattern foreseen by Swales in the model above?
3) Write a first draft of the introduction in your target language based on the moves you have identified.

Why is an understanding of moves useful for the translator?

Firstly, moves are organizational tools shared by most of the languages which translators in this field will work with. As far as drafting is concerned, what matters is the move itself – that is, the kind of information it contains and the function it fulfils in the overall structure of the text – and not the particular form in which it is expressed in the source language. In fact, if we focus only on the linguistic details of the source text and ignore the progression of moves we may miss key organizational patterns on which coherence and cohesion are built.

Secondly, they give us a broader view of text progression beyond terminology. They can alert us to the need for signposting, which will help our reader to process the target text. It is particularly useful to focus on common genres (see chapter 2) and to learn how to navigate the well-used channels down which the message flows.

Thirdly, since they are recurrent patterns, familiarity with them allows us to predict with a fair degree of confidence: a) what the likely structure will be; b) the linguistic resources in the target language most likely to be appropriate for each of the elements making up the whole pattern; and c) possible difficulties which may occur.

Fourthly, recognition of these patterns allows us to move more freely in the text and avoid a linear approach to writing when needed.

Finally, familiarity with these patterns eventually makes conscious translation decisions become habits, thus speeding the process up.

Task 7. Drafting structured abstracts

Here is a version of an abstract of an original article published by New England Journal of Medicine from which the headings have been removed.

1) Read it carefully.
2) Decide how the text should be distributed under these heading: 'Background', 'Methods', 'Results', 'Conclusions'.
3) Write a structured draft of it in your target language using these four headings.
4) Check your choice of structure against the real one published at <http://content.nejm.org/cgi/content/short/344/13/967>. You can also access the real summary at Medline <http://www.ncbi.nlm.nih.gov/entrez> simply by typing the title in inverted commas into the search engine.

Preventing Recurrent Upper Gastrointestinal Bleeding in Patients with Helicobacter pylori Infection Who Are Taking Low-Dose Aspirin or Naproxen

Many patients who have had upper gastrointestinal bleeding continue to take low-dose aspirin for cardiovascular prophylaxis or other nonsteroidal anti-inflammatory drugs (NSAIDs) for musculoskeletal pain. It is uncertain whether infection with *Helicobacter pylori* is a risk factor for bleeding in such patients. We studied patients with a history of upper gastrointestinal bleeding who were infected with *H. pylori* and who were taking low-dose aspirin or other NSAIDs. We evaluated whether eradication of the infection or omeprazole treatment was more effective in preventing recurrent bleeding. We recruited patients who presented with upper gastrointestinal bleeding that was confirmed by endoscopy. Their ulcers were healed by daily treatment with 20 mg of omeprazole for eight weeks or longer. Then, those who had been taking aspirin were given 80 mg of aspirin daily, and those who had been taking other NSAIDs were given 500 mg of naproxen twice daily for six months. The patients in each group were then randomly assigned separately to receive 20 mg of omeprazole daily for six months or one week of eradication therapy, consisting of 120 mg of bismuth subcitrate, 500 mg of tetracycline, and 400 mg of metronidazole, all given four times daily, followed by placebo for six months. We enrolled 400 patients (250 of whom were taking aspirin and 150 of whom were taking other NSAIDs). Among those taking aspirin, the probability of recurrent bleeding during the six-month period was 1.9 percent for patients who received eradication therapy and 0.9 percent for patients who received omeprazole (absolute difference, 1.0 percent; 95 percent confidence interval for the difference, −1.9 to 3.9 percent). Among users of other NSAIDs, the probability of recurrent bleeding was 18.8 percent for patients receiving eradication therapy and 4.4 percent for those treated with omeprazole (absolute difference, 14.4 percent; 95 percent confidence interval for the difference, 4.4 to 24.4 percent; P=0.005). Among patients with *H. pylori* infection and a history of upper gastrointestinal bleeding who are taking low-dose aspirin, the eradication of *H. pylori* is equivalent to treatment with omeprazole in preventing recurrent bleeding. Omeprazole is superior to the eradication of *H. pylori* in preventing recurrent bleeding in patients who are taking other NSAIDs, such as naproxen.

Signalling moves in argumentation

Now we move on to argumentation, a complex rhetorical operation the purpose of which is to persuade and convince. These are typical in the biomedical and health sectors: a research team wanting to convince the readers of the relevance, validity and truth of their results; a health organization trying to make the general public aware of the importance of preventing a particular disease; a medical association trying to advise health professionals about the efficacy of using a specific procedure or drug; and so forth.

One of the main difficulties in the translation of an argument is that it is not always overt. The other is that it does not take place locally − that is, within the limits of one sentence or a small group of sentences – but may take place throughout the text.

For example, in an original article we find different strategies to convince the reader of the relevance, validity and truth of what is said:

- Authority from respected persons and institutions. This is reflected in the text in the form of citation, allusions, and so forth (**intertextual strategies**)
- Data, results, methods to get the data, and so forth (**empirical strategies**)
- Critical analysis, common sense, logical reasoning, deduction, inference, and so forth (**interpretative strategies**)

Hatim and Mason (1997: 192) have pointed out above mentioned difficulties when translating arguments: 'In the translation of argumentation, translators more often than not find themselves operating with greater degrees of latitude than those commonly offered by instruction and exposition.' Exploring moves and using them to draft the target text may help you deal better with those greater degrees of latitude mentioned by Hatim and Mason. For example, sometimes it can be sensible to rearrange the different steps of the argumentation so as to make a stronger case.

Paradis and Zimmerman (1997:37) have established a basic five-move pattern of argumentation in scientific and technical texts that can be used as a general starting point for our drafting purposes:

1. A problem or situation to be remedied
2. A claim or thesis that resolves the problem
3. Background issues that give the particulars of the problem and establish criteria for solving it
4. Evidence that supports the claim or thesis that applies the criteria
5. A discussion in which the evidence is weighed and shown to support the claim

Now let's have a look at a real example. The following paragraph is the last paragraph of a report in which the authors give advice about the use of vitamin E in the prevention of heart disease:

> In view of these findings, the most prudent and scientifically supportable recommendation for the general population is to consume a balanced diet with emphasis on antioxidant-rich fruits and vegetables and whole grains. This advice, which is consistent with the current dietary guidelines of the American Heart Association, considers the role of the total diet in influencing disease risk. Although diet alone may not provide the levels of vitamin E intake that have been associated with the lowest risk in a

few observational studies, the absence of efficacy and safety data from randomized trials precludes the establishment of population-wide recommendations regarding vitamin E supplementation.

We can see that this particular argumentation is based on several moves that could be summarized in the following sequence:

1. Recommendation
2. Supporting the recommendation
3. Limitations of the recommendation
4. Rejecting another potential recommendation
5. Reasons for rejecting the other potential recommendation

Task 8. Composing an argumentation through moves

1) Read the text about the use of vitamin E again.
2) Without looking at the English text, answer in your target language the following questions based on the five-move pattern: a) What is recommended? b) Why should we rely on it? c) What are its limitations? d) What other potential recommendation must be rejected? e) Why?
3) Without looking at the English text, write a draft of the above paragraph in your target language that clearly reflects this five-move pattern.

Go to *British Medical Journal,* vol. 326, 10 May 2003 <http://bmj.com> and find the article entitled 'Association between antidepressant prescribing and suicide in Australia, 1991-2000: trend analysis'. Look now at the structure of the discussion section. The point of the argument is: Is there is a causal relationship between antidepressant prescribing and suicide decrease? If so, how strong is it? The argument is particularly fuzzy in this case presumably because the authors are being very cautious. In order to provide a more convincing argument, the authors of the study include these two subsections:

- **Excluding possible alternative explanations**, in which they present other possible explanations that the reader might think of, such as unemployment or alcohol consumption, and give evidence to reject them.
- **Positive evidence for causal interpretation**, in which they present other explanations that support the hypothesis that antidepressant prescribing does have a positive effect on the reduction of suicide rates.

Recognizing these types of moves, their communicative purpose and the way they are linguistically realized is particularly relevant when composing arguments in the 'Discussion' section of original articles and other related genres.

Task 9. Completing an argumentation in your target language

1) Go to *British Medical Journal,* vol. 326, 10 May 2003 <http://bmj. com> and find the article entitled 'Association between antidepressant prescribing and suicide in Australia, 1991-2000: trend analysis'.
2) Read carefully the subsection 'Excluding possible alternative explana- tions' in the 'Discussion'.
3) Complete both columns of the table below in your target language.

Possible explanation	*Reason for rejection*
1) Suicide is under-reported	
2)	
3) Unemployment	
4)	
5) Improvement in quality of life	

The methodology presented in this chapter can be used in the drafting of common medical genres, such as patient information leaflets, clinical trial protocols, stan- dard operating procedures, case reports, and informed consents (see chapter 2).

Some practical reminders and suggestions when composing the target text:

- What you are producing at this stage is only a draft. Don't get side- tracked by small details; you will sort them out later. Concentrate on the flow of ideas, on the main elements of the narration, descrip- tion or argumentation. What really matters now is that you map the overall structure and content of the target text.
- Write the headings of all sections and subsections first. Then draft the part that seems easiest to you, regardless of whether it is the first one. Write around missing information if necessary. Leave the title until the end.
- Draft the main idea of the text, wherever this may occur, and then continue hierarchically from most to least important, regardless of the linear order.

- Re-read the source text as many times as you need to in order to identify hierarchy and types of information.
- When writing the outline and developing it further, pay special attention to the different types of information contained in each section as well as to their function and communicative purpose. The target text should contain the appropriate type of information in the right place; if necessary, move information from one section to another or rearrange it within the same section.
- In-house style norms in the target context may affect the structure of the text; make sure you know and observe them when outlining your target text.
- The structure of a particular genre may vary from language to language; use parallel texts to find out possible differences.
- The structure may not be indicated by headings and subheadings; pay attention to moves and work from them.
- Moves do not necessarily coincide with paragraphs and do not necessarily follow the same order in texts of the same genre.
- In some genres, moves are fixed and regular; in other genres (e.g. scientific editorials) authors have greater freedom and the moves depend on their preferences.
- Try to recognize move structure in genres with which you are not familiar and retain the pattern in your mind.
- Watch out for differences in move structure of the same genre in different languages.

4.4 Crafting your target text

Now we leave macroelements in order to focus on microelements and deal with more local aspects of text production such as linking, titling, paragraphing, emphasizing and hedging, and wording. By crafting we mean the way in which writers and translators put together the various pieces of the text, linking ideas through sentences and paragraphs within an overall structure.

Imagine yourself translating the following paragraph (example taken from Matthews et al, 2000: 108):

> Two canine cadavers with orthopaedic abnormalities were identified which included a first dog that had an unusual deformity secondary to premature closure of the distal ulnar physis and a second dog that had a hypertrophic nonunion of the femur, and the radius and femur of both dogs were harvested and cleaned of soft tissue.

You decide to render it in your mother tongue following the same syntactic pattern, that is, all in one sentence. As a result, you've got the factual content in your target text, but you may not be satisfied with the excessive length of the sentence and decide to split it up into several sentences. This could be a gloss of your target text:

> Two canine cadavers with orthopaedic abnormalities were identified. The first dog had an unusual deformity. It was secondary to premature closure of the distal ulnar physis. The second dog had a hypertrophic nonunion of the femur. The radius and femur of both dogs were harvested. They were cleaned of soft tissue.

Now you have probably gone too far. The sentences are too short and the whole paragraph sounds very fragmented and abrupt. You need to recraft it so that the target text reads more smoothly, and your reader feels more comfortable:

> Two canine cadavers with orthopaedic abnormalities were identified. The first dog had an unusual deformity secondary to premature closure of the distal ulnar physis; the second, a hypertrophic nonunion of the femur. The radius and femur of both dogs were harvested and cleaned of soft tissue.

This third recrafting not only reads better but also is slightly shorter than the previous ones. Although the order of presentation of the information has not been altered, it has been reconnected in a different way by means of changes at sentence level, which affect punctuation and cohesion.

Paragraphing

Imagine you were faced with a long text in which there were no paragraphs. How would you feel? Why would a text with paragraphs be preferable? What, then, does paragraphing do?

Well, of course, it helps us to navigate the text by breaking it down into more manageable chunks. The beginnings of paragraphs usually link logically with the previous paragraphs while their ends move us along, preparing us for the ideas to come. These links act as signposts for readers and save them mental effort. So, as we draft the target text, we should pay attention to three key aspects: 1) position of paragraph within the whole section or text; 2) links with the paragraph before and the paragraph after; and 3) internal order of the paragraph.

Paradis and Zimmerman (1997: 51) state: 'Commonly, each paragraph is linked with the preceding paragraph, makes some kind of generalization or claim in a topic sentence, and then develops this claim in a series of supporting sentences.'

If this is the case in our source text, then there is no need for us to alter the paragraph in the target text. But more often than not, we need to adjust paragraph length and distribution so as to make the target text smoother and more readable. Have a look at the following paragraph, which could be a gloss of a translation into your target language:

> A) Depression is a risk factor for suicide, and antidepressants reduce suicidal ideation. There is little direct evidence that antidepressants reduce the suicide rate because suicide is rare even among clinically depressed people, and even large clinical trials of antidepressants have had limited power to detect a reduction. Nonetheless, there is reasonable epidemiological evidence that antidepressants reduce suicide rates in depressed patients. But there are more reasons for believing that increased antidepressant prescribing may have contributed to the decline in suicide, as for example, the fact that the prescription of antidepressant drugs is also often accompanied by other assessments (such as asking about suicide risk, giving information to family members) and clinical interventions (counselling, support, ongoing clinical review). These interventions, in combination with medication, may reduce suicidal behaviour.

Now compare it with the following recrafting:

> B) There are several reasons for believing that increased antidepressant prescribing may have contributed to the decline in suicide. Firstly, depression is a risk factor for suicide, and antidepressants reduce suicidal ideation. There is little direct evidence that antidepressants reduce the suicide rate because suicide is rare even among clinically depressed people, and even large clinical trials of antidepressants have had limited power to detect a reduction. Nonetheless, there is reasonable epidemiological evidence that antidepressants reduce suicide rates in depressed patients.
>
> Secondly, the prescription of antidepressant drugs is also often accompanied by other assessments (such as asking about suicide risk, giving information to family members) and clinical interventions (counselling, support, ongoing clinical review). These interventions, in combination with medication, may reduce suicidal behaviour.

In the reworked version (B), we have identified the topic idea, have expressed it clearly, have put it right at the beginning of the paragraph, and have signalled the supporting ideas by means of 'Firstly' and 'Secondly'. Furthermore, we have divided the paragraph into two different ones making them lighter and reflecting the logic of the enumeration.

This makes it easier for readers to follow the argument because they don't have to construct it themselves, as they would in the first version.

Linking

Once paragraphs are well connected with one another and ordered internally, flow within the paragraph is a key element for successful communication.

In the following example we have deleted four linking words or phrases. Translate the text into your mother tongue completing the missing linking words.

> Systematic errors in the data on suicide or antidepressants may have biased the results. Suicides, ..., are under-reported, and there are likely to be errors in using general practice prescription profiles to estimate sex and age differences in use from sales data. It is unlikely, ..., that under-reporting of suicide should have changed over time or that such under-reporting, or any errors in the general practice survey data, would both vary by age and sex in the ways required to explain the patterns in our data.
>
> Trends in risk factors for suicide, ... unemployment and per capita alcohol consumption, may explain the decline in suicide. Per capita alcohol consumption (calculated from sales data) shows a substantial decline in the early 1990s in Australia, ... it remained steady throughout the remainder of the 1990s. This was mirrored by trends in alcohol related injuries.

You can check your linking words with those in the original text by going to *British Medical Journal,* vol. 326, 10 May 2003 <http://bmj.com> and find the article entitled 'Association between antidepressant prescribing and suicide in Australia, 1991-2000: trend analysis'.

> It is important for you to have a rich and varied repertoire of linking words and phrases in your mother tongue to express a variety of functions such as addition ('furthermore', 'what's more', 'moreover', 'besides'), adversativity ('although', 'however', 'nevertheless', 'all the same', 'even though'), cause and effect ('as a consequence', 'consequently', 'therefore', 'as a result', 'thus', 'hence'), clarification ('in other words', 'that is'), contrast ('while', 'whereas', 'on the contrary'), or illustration ('for example', 'for instance').

Linking words and phrases are not the only cohesive devices. In the examples which follow, we provide some possible glosses of a translation of a scientific paper. Read them carefully and decide which of the two in each pair reads better, and why.

> 1a) Some dietary recommendations aim at reducing the risk of coronary heart disease. They have focused largely on the intake of nutrients that

affect established risk factors. Among those nutrients we find plasma lipid and lipoprotein levels, blood pressure, and body weight.
1b) Dietary recommendations aimed at reducing the risk of coronary heart disease have focused largely on the intake of nutrients that affect established risk factors, including plasma lipid and lipoprotein levels, blood pressure, and body weight.

2a) Recent developments in our understanding of the atherosclerotic process and factors that trigger ischemic events have led to the consideration of dietary constituents that may alter risk through other mechanisms.
2b) The consideration of dietary constituents that may alter risk through other mechanisms comes from recent developments in our understanding of the atherosclerotic process and factors that trigger ischemic events have led to.

3a) Prominent among these are antioxidants. Antioxidants are proposed to inhibit multiple proatherogenic and prothrombotic oxidative events in the artery wall.
3b) Prominent among these are antioxidants, which are proposed to inhibit multiple proatherogenic and prothrombotic oxidative events in the artery wall.

4a) This report provides a brief overview of evidence concerning a role for dietary antioxidants in disease prevention. It places emphasis on studies in human populations. It describes a number of issues that should be resolved before it would be prudent to make recommendations regarding the prophylactic use of antioxidant supplements.
4b) This report provides a brief overview of evidence concerning a role for dietary antioxidants in disease prevention, with emphasis on studies in human populations, and describes a number of issues that should be resolved before it would be prudent to make recommendations regarding the prophylactic use of antioxidant supplements.

Back referencing

When crafting the target text, it is important to link its parts so that it moves on in a coherent way. Have a look at these two examples and compare the edited original and the possible gloss of the translation:

> *Edited original:* 'This notion opened the way for connecting the fabric of social and cultural phenomena to specific features of neurobiology, which is supported by powerful facts.'
> *Gloss of the TT:* 'This notion opened the way for connecting the fabric of social and cultural phenomena to specific features of neurobiology, a

connection supported by powerful facts.'

Connecting → connection

Edited original: 'Suicides, for example, are under-reported, and there are likely to be errors in using general practice prescription profiles to estimate sex and age differences in use from sales data. It is unlikely, however, that it should have changed over time or it, or any errors in the general practice survey data, would both vary by age and sex in the ways required to explain the patterns in our data.'

Gloss of the TT: 'Suicides, for example, are under-reported, and there are likely to be errors in using general practice prescription profiles to estimate sex and age differences in use from sales data. It is unlikely, however, that under-reporting of suicide should have changed over time or that such under-reporting, or any errors in the general practice survey data, would both vary by age and sex in the ways required to explain the patterns in our data.'

Suicides are under-reported → under-reporting of suicide.

In these two examples back reference has been reinforced in the target text by means of nominalizations: 'connecting' becomes 'connection', and 'suicides are under-reported' becomes 'under-reporting of suicide', thus reinforcing coherence, clarity, readability, and smoothness. Note that in the edited original on two occasions the word 'it' is inadequate as it is not clear what refers to. In the gloss this problem has been resolved.

There are other ways of referring back unambiguously to something already mentioned: repetition of a word; replacing a noun with a pronoun; using a synonym or paraphrase; using an antonym; using a comparison; or using an adverbial reference.

Emphasizing and hedging

Let's focus now on one of the most important pragmatic aspects when crafting the target text. By hedging we mean the fact that a statement is not presented categorically, thus reducing the writer's commitment to the truth of the propositions. Both emphasizing and hedging have to do with the attitude and point of view of the writer. Notice them in the following examples:

1. '*Remember*: this medicine is for you. *Only* a doctor can prescribe it for you. *Never* give this medicine to anyone else'.
2. 'The needle *must* be inserted in an intercostal space overlying the fluid'.

3. 'But placebos *may* also have adverse effects, including nausea, dizziness, sleepiness, insomnia, fatigue, depression, numbness, hallucinations, itching, vomiting, tremor, tachycardia, diarrhoea, pallor, rashes, hives, ataxia, and edema.'
4. 'Since Ermakova's unique study was small and not yet peer-reviewed, we *cannot* fairly draw any conclusions as to if or how Roundup Ready soy influences offspring. From what we *do* know about GM soy, however, *there are* several ways in which it *might* influence the health of the next generation'.

The information contained in the source text is seldom presented in a neutral, detached, flat way. As they communicate knowledge to the readers, authors also express their attitudes not only towards their readers but also towards the contents and ideas they want to communicate. Sometimes they want to emphasize a point – as in examples 1 and 2 – whereas at other times they need to be cautious about what they are saying – as in example 3. In some other cases – such as example 4 – we find a complex combination of caution (hedging) and emphasis. In these four examples we find modal expressions that reflect the author's attitude of emphasis or/and caution towards the readers and the contents.

Modality is one of the main ways of expressing emphasis and caution. It is a gradable phenomenon through which we can express different degrees of certainty and obligation:

- Impossible – possible – necessary/certain
- Forbidden – permitted – obligatory

Modality, however, is not restricted to modal verbs (such as 'must', 'can', 'may', 'might'), but includes a variety of linguistic resources, such as adverbs ('probably', 'presumably', 'surely', 'definitely', 'evidently', 'supposedly', 'undoubtedly', 'certainly'), adjectives ('likely', 'probable', 'possible', 'reasonable', 'significant', 'clear', 'obvious', 'self-evident'), main verbs ('suggest', 'point', 'appear', 'seem', 'show', 'indicate', 'demonstrate') and expressions ('on the whole', 'in the main', 'in general', 'with some exceptions', 'as it is generally assumed', 'in our opinion', 'as far as we know', 'to our knowledge').

We find one of the richest and most productive areas of modality in biomedical texts in the expression of cause-and-effect relationships, as can be seen in the following examples:

- 'Parenteral iron *provokes* oxidative stress in patients with CKD (chronic kidney disease).'
- 'Antiretroviral drugs used in the treatment of HIV infection have been *associated* with many hematologic toxicities, which are more common in patients with advanced disease.'
- 'During normal aging, the lens of the eye becomes thicker, *resulting* in in-

creased apposition between the pupillary margin and the lens.'
- **'Actinic keratoses** are precancerous keratotic lesions that are a frequent, disturbing *consequence* of many years of sun exposure.'
- 'Rasmussen encephalitis (RE) is a rare devastating disease of childhood *causing* progressive neurological deficits and intractable seizures, typically affecting one hemisphere.'
- 'Wilson disease (WD) is a rare inborn copper storage disease *leading to* liver cirrhosis and neuropsychological deterioration.'
- 'Rabbit ischemic myocardial injury was *induced* by occluding the anterior descent of the left artery (LAD).'
- 'We found a *significant association* between medication compliance and substance abuse (OR 0.52, CI 0.32-0.85), involuntary admission (OR 0.60, CI 0.41-0.89), history of aggressive behavior (OR 0.57, CI 0.38-0.85), and no school graduation (OR 0.59, CI 0.41-0.86).'
- 'Reduced access to insulin-sensitive tissues in dogs with obesity *secondary* to increased fat intake.'
- 'Studies on the nature of at least some satellite cells, including their capabilities for self-renewal and for *giving rise* to multiple lineages in a stem cell-like function, are exploring the molecular basis of phenotypes described by markers of specialized function and gene expression in normal development, neuromuscular disease and aging.'
- 'Reactive oxygen species have been implicated in the *etiology* of multiple organ dyspepsia syndrome and infection's complications in patients with trauma.'

This variety and richness in the expression of different degrees of emphasis and hedging as far as cause-and-effect relationships are concerned is especially important when crafting the target text. The same should be said about any other expression of attitude towards the readers and the contents by means of modality.

Task 10. Dealing with different degrees of causal relationships

1) Read the eleven sentences above and order them from the strongest to the weakest as far as cause-and-effect relationships are con cerned.
2) Decide which of them express the same causal degree; in other words, which of them are interchangeable in the contexts in which they appear.
3) Translate them into your mother tongue paying special attention to the italicized words or expressions.

> 4) In order to understand the sentences better, find the contexts in which they appear by going to <http://www.ncbi.nlm.nih.gov/ Da tabase/index. html>.
>
> 5) Find other ways of expressing different degrees of causal relationships in medical texts written in your target language.

Wording

When crafting the target text we must pay attention not only to the content that we communicate but also to the preferred expressions used to communicate it – also referred to as phraseology or prefabricated expressions. In medical genres there are preferred ways of saying things. Have a look at the following expressions taken from a PIL (see chapter 2):

- 'Keep this leaflet. You may need to read it again.'
- 'If you have further questions, please ask your doctor or your pharmacist.'
- 'Keep all medicines out of reach of children.'
- 'Do not exceed stated dose.'

The phraseology of some parts of the SPC (Summary of product characteristics) is also highly conventionalized.

- 'X causes/is thought to cause serious birth defects when administered during pregnancy.'
- 'X is contraindicated in pregnancy.'
- 'X has harmful pharmacological effects on pregnancy and/or the foetus/ newborn child.'
- 'For X no clinical data on exposed pregnancies are available.'
- 'Well-conducted epidemiological studies indicate no adverse effects of X on pregnancy or on the health of the foetus/newborn child. X can be used during pregnancy.'
- 'The concomitant medication X adversely interacts with oral contraceptives (OCs). Therefore an alternative, effective and safe method of contraception should be used during (and up to x weeks after) treatment.'

Task 11. Dealing with preferred wordings in medical genres

1) Translate the above sentences into your mother tongue.
2) Check your translation in published parallel texts (see EMEA's site for translations in several European languages)

Collocations − preferred combination of words − are equally important when crafting the text. For example, in biomedical abstracts published in English the adverb 'postoperatively' tends to appear, on the one hand, with the noun 'patients' and, on the other hand, with the verbs 'explore', 'diagnose', 'assess', 'perform', 'analyze', 'administer', 'interview', and 'premedicate' in sentences such as:

- 'Blood samples drawn from 44 patients with breast cancer were *preoperatively* analyzed [...]'
- 'A neuropsychological test battery (9 tests) was administered *preoperatively* [...]'
- 'PTH (Parathyroid hormone) levels were measured *preoperatively* and 30 minutes postoperatively.'

Thus the lexical combination of 'postoperatively' + 'patient' + one of the above mentioned verbs constitutes a preferred way of wording − mainly in passive sentences − in research genres written in English.

To make the target text fully adequate and acceptable, we must discover collocational patterns in our target language. This can be done intuitively after many years of conscious practice or by means of automatic lexical analyzers such as Wordsmith Tools (for further information on this tool, go to <http://www.lexically.net/wordsmith>.

Finally, medical writers have a repertoire of prefabricated expressions that they use for different rhetorical purposes, such as supporting their interests, referring to previous research without bothering to review and summarize it, validating their results, acknowledging help from colleagues, and so forth. In the following table, Matthews et al (1996, 2000: 104) reproduce a humorous interpretation of this sort of common expressions in biomedical research genres:

What the scientist said	*What the scientist meant*
It has long been known that...	I haven't bothered to look up the original reference, but...
Of great theoretical importance...	Interesting to me...
Typical results are shown...	The best results are shown...
It is suggested that; It is believed that; It may be that...	I think...
It is generally believed that...	A couple of other guys think so, too.

It is clear that much additional work will be required before a complete understanding....	I don't understand it.
Unfortunately, a quantitative theory to account for these results has not been formulated.	I can't think of one, and neither can anyone else.
Correct within an order of magnitude.	Wrong.
Thanks are due to Joe Clotz for assistance with experiments and to Boyton Fird for valuable discussion.	Clotz did the work, and Fird interpreted the data.

Figure 4.9. Prefabricated expressions in research genres:
a humorous view

Titling

We all know that titles (and subtitles) are used to give readers an idea of what is to follow, so that after glancing at the title they have a good idea of whether they want to read on or not. Titles, thus, save the readers time if they are not interested, but if they are, help to prepare them mentally for what they are about to read. They may already at this stage have certain expectations about possible arguments, structure, terminology, and so forth.

When drafting the title of the target text we should take into account two aspects: the overall communicative purpose of the title and its structure.

There are two kinds of titles as far as communicative purpose is concerned: a) those which tell us what a paper is about (indicative); and b) those which sum up in one sentence the main message of the paper (informative). Have a look at the following examples:

Type of title	*Examples*
a) Indicative	Mouse Models of Diabetic Nephropathy
b) Informative	Biliverdin therapy protects rat livers from ischemia and reperfusion injury

Figure 4.10. Types of titles according to their function

As far as the structure of titles is concerned, Huth (1999: 132) has posited three types: a) a single continuous title; b) a title with subordinate terms following a colon; and c) a title and a subtitle. He offers the following examples of each:

Type of structure	Examples
a) A single continuous title	Transplants of Umbilical-Cord Blood or Bone Marrow from Unrelated Donors in Adults with Acute Leukemia
b) A title with subordinate terms following a colon	Differentiation of Mesenchymal Stem Cells Towards a Nucleus Pulposus-like Phenotype In Vitro: Implications for Cell-Based Transplantation Therapy
c) A title and a subtitle	A Carboxypeptidase Inhibitor from the tick Rhipicephalus bursa. Isolation, cDNA cloning, recombinant expression, and characterization

Figure 4.11. Types of titles according to their structure

Task 12. Drafting titles

1) Go to *PubMed* at <http://www.ncbi.nlm.nih.gov/entrez/query.fcgi>.
2) Enter any medical term in the search engine.
3) Without reading the title, choose an abstract and read it carefully.
4) Draft an indicative title for that abstract either in English or in your target language.
5) Draft an informative title for the same abstract either in English or in your target language.
6) Read the original title and compare it with the two titles you have drafted.

It may seem strange that titling is the last thing we are considering, when the title of a text always appears at the very beginning. The reason for this is that it is often a waste of time to write the title before you write the body of your target text because frequently what you chose in advance will turn out to be inappropriate.

Some practical reminders and suggestions when crafting the target text:

• Divide excessively long paragraphs at logical points.

- Look at how the closing sentence of a paragraph and the first sentence of the next one are connected.
- Check each paragraph to see whether its general sequence moves along a clear line of thought.
- Avoid unnecessary ambiguity by linking appropriately the different parts of the sentence or paragraph.
- Make connections between or within sentences explicit when necessary.
- Adjust the degree of emphasis and hedging so as to accurately reflect the writer's attitude towards both the readers and the content of the text.
- Make sure that the combinations of words you use are idiomatic.
- Make sure you use the standard translation of prefabricated expressions in highly conventionalized genres.
- Consider changing the communicative purpose of the title if it fits the assignment better.
- Consider changing the structure of the title if it fits the assignment better.
- Avoid abbreviations in titles.
- Make sure that the title contains the key words in the text.
- Try to place the most important key words at the beginning.
- Check the title once you have translated the rest of the text so as to ensure terminological consistency.
- Make the title as succinct as possible.

4.5 Improving the draft

Once you have composed the overall structure and crafted the contents of each of the parts of the target text, it is time to sort out any details, both conceptual and formal, that have not yet been addressed.

Conceptual and terminological accuracy is one of the key elements in medical translation since the value of the text often lies in its factual content. Hence, in professional practice a great deal of the working time at this stage is spent on terminological issues such as fully understanding the exact sense of particular terms and making adjustments to the target text so that the reader is not misled; making sure that complex concepts and the relationship between them are fully understandable in the target text; finding just the right term in the target language, especially in cases of terminological mismatch; finding sound solutions in cases of neologisms; exploring synonyms in the target language and deciding which is more suitable for a particular target text; making sure that terminological solutions are consistent throughout the target text; and detecting and sorting out false synonyms and false friends. These writing tasks often involve considerable time spent researching and consulting reliable information sources (see chapter 6), mainly dictionaries, terminological databases and textbooks about the specific subject matter. They also involve knowledge about terminological variation, especially criteria to sort out neologisms (see chapter 7).

Ideally, of course, a translation should read like an original text, that is, the readers should not be aware that they are reading a translation. It should feel absolutely right. So what, exactly, would make us suspect that we are dealing with a translation? Clearly, gross grammatical, lexical and syntactic errors would render the translation unfit for its purpose – whatever that purpose might be. But there are other, subtler infelicities which might make the reader slightly uncomfortable because the text does not ring quite true. These might involve the nearly-but-not-quite-suitable choice of lexis, word order, verb form, deixis, or a very slightly unexpected presentation of elements within a very slightly unexpected structural framework. In other words, the failure to conform to all the norms expected by readers – and the fact that this will tend to slow down their processing of the text – means that instead of a good translation, we might have one that is just about adequate or even unacceptable.

Becoming aware of norms

In addition to conceptual and terminological accuracy, for a translation to be fully acceptable and accepted – both as a functional text and as a representation of the target culture – it has to conform to the explicit and implicit norms (regularities, conventions, expectations, habits, preferences) that regulate written communication in the target situation. The following facts are especially relevant to the medical translator:

- Different professional communities (nurses, pharmacists, pharmacologists, physiotherapists, psychologists, surgeons, GPs, physicians, researchers) tend to have different norms as far as the use of medical language is concerned. For example, the way nurses and physicians explain the same disease to a patient will vary in degree of detail and depth since they see it from different perspectives and use the information for different purposes.
- Research journals may have different norms as far as structure and length of texts, terminology, spelling and style are concerned. For example, one journal may require structured abstracts whereas another may ask for non-structured abstracts.
- Publishing houses, pharmaceutical laboratories and health organizations normally have different in-house style norms.
- Medical specialties may have different norms as far as terminology is concerned. For example, the same anatomical part may be referred to in different

ways in descriptive anatomy (Latin name) and in sports physiotherapy (popular name).

- Health systems in different countries have different norms as far as information
  policies and patient status are concerned. For example, in private health
  systems, the patient is a client and is treated as such. In some countries the
  language used in written communication with patients is more explicit than
  in others owing to possible legal consequences.

- Different cultures may have different norms in the communication of medical
  information. For example, in more literate cultures written medical communication is carried out in highly conventionalized genres, whereas in oral
  societies medical communication takes a very different form.

- Different genres are ruled by different norms as far as register, tenor,
  terminology, modality, and style are concerned. For example, the patient
  information leaflet of a specific drug uses a far more personal tenor than the
  corresponding summary of product characteristics for the same drug. You may
  be extremely accurate when dealing with the concepts and terms related to
  a particular drug, but if you are not well aware of the pragmatic and formal
  differences between a summary of product characteristics and a patient information leaflet for that same drug you may easily mistranslate your text.

When dealing with medical translation assignments we discover that norms can
be both explicit and implicit. Explicit norms are visible, easy to identify and
to observe. For example, the in-house style sheet for authors of a specialized
journal contains explicit norms that can easily be followed in the writing of the
target text.

But implicit norms may not be so visible. Variations in the use of tenses, tenor,
passive voice or nominalization are not made explicit and may be more difficult
to detect and to observe.

Detecting formal variations and conforming to norms

In the previous section we have dealt with all kinds of differences in a variety of
contexts that may affect decisions in the writing of the target text. Now we will
focus on formal variations resulting from the different ways genres are ruled by
different norms. We can establish three types of variation:

- The same genre can present variations of structure, register, terminology, tenor,
  style, modality and so on in different languages. This is one of the things the
  medical translator frequently has to deal with. For example, in original articles
  published in English hedging – the use of modal devices to express caution
  – is more frequently used than in original articles published in Spanish.
- Two texts that deal with exactly the same topic in the same language but which

belong to different genres may present variations of style, tenor, modality, use of verbal tenses, treatment of terminology, and so on. This is also relevant to medical translators (see chapter 2), especially when dealing with genre shifts (see next section).

- Different parts of the same genre in the same language may present all kinds of formal variations. This is particularly important when polishing the final version of the target text. For example, the use of personal pronouns and passive voice often varies between sections in original articles in English.

Study of parallel texts (see chapter 6) is the main tool for detecting genre variations which are relevant to the finishing of the target text. The study of parallel texts can be done manually or automatically by means of text analyzers.

Use bias-free, inclusive language

People suffering from certain diseases may be particularly sensitive to the language used to refer to them and their illnesses. We must beware of using biased language and unacceptable labels. Even certain euphemisms may fall out of favour and cause offence. Such labels change rapidly and we need to keep up-to-date with what is currently acceptable.

There may be various reasons why a source text has been written in biased, exclusive language such as lack of awareness and sensitivity on the part of the author, or their social context. However, the fact that the source text uses biased, exclusive language does not mean that we must also use it in the target text. The following recommendation made to medical writers by Matthews et al (2000: 151-154) can also be made to translators:

- *Specify only the differences that are relevant*
  Differences such as sexual orientation, marital status, age, ethnic identity, or the fact that a person has a disability should be mentioned only when relevant.
- *Be sensitive to group labels*
  Labels such as 'the schizophrenic' vs 'the normal' in the context of a clinical study may stigmatize individuals with differences. In these cases, we should avoid the label and use a more descriptive solution in the target text, such as 'people diagnosed with schizophrenia' in the above example.
- *Guard against the perception of bias or prejudice*
  Racism and sexism are two of the most frequent types of prejudice. They may or may not be conscious or intentional. Furthermore, the situation varies in different languages, cultures, and countries. Whereas in some there is more awareness and respect, in others there is more tolerance to sexism

and racism. As translators, we should find alternatives and avoid racist and sexist language whether it be unconscious and unintentional or 'normal' in a given language, culture or country.

- *Avoid awkward coinage*
  In the effort to avoid racism and sexism in our target text we may go too far and end up sounding artificial and ridiculous. A middle ground is often preferable so as to avoid undesirable effects.

Finishing the final draft

There comes a point when, whether we like it or not, we have to finish the assignment and deliver it to the client. There is always time pressure in professional practice. Deadlines are short and things have to get done. In fact, our professional credibility depends not only on the quality of the target text but also on meeting deadlines. At this stage, inexperienced translators in particular may be plagued by doubts and uncertainties about the quality of what they are about to deliver as the finished product. One thought that should comfort us is that we are not asked to do *the* perfect translation of a particular text. We receive an assignment and the quality of the target text depends both on the terms of the assignment, and, the purpose or function of the translation.

The quality required in a text that will be published is not the same as that needed for a text that will be used internally by a few readers and for a limited period of time. Thus we should establish the difference between what *can* be improved and what *should* be improved in a specific assignment. In other words, nearly every thing in a translation can be improved. Even if it is perfectly correct and adequate, the best translation can be questioned and improved on the grounds of personal taste. But in professional translation what really matters are improvements which will eliminate errors or inadequacies, and meet the quality requirements of the task.

Five different areas should be taken into account:

- Coherence between the source text and the target text
- Coherence within the target text
- Terminology
- Grammar and style
- Formal presentation

The following questions explore these five areas of interest and may help to decide what *can* and what really *should* be improved in a particular assignment before it is completely finished:

- Coherence between the source text and the target text
  - Does the translation reflect the intended meaning of the source text? (Accuracy)
  - Have any of the factual elements of the message been left out without justification? (Completeness)

- Coherence within the target text
  - Does the sequence of ideas make sense; is there any nonsense or contradiction? (Logic)
  - Are there any factual, conceptual or mathematical errors? (Facts)

- Terminology
  - Is terminology unified throughout the text? Are there misleading synonyms? (Consistency)
  - Does it reflect the preferences of the client and the target genre? (Tailoring)

- Grammar and style
  - Does the text flow? Are the connections between sentences clear? Are the relationships among the parts of each sentence clear? Are there any awkward, hard-to-read sentences? (Smoothness)
  - Is the style suited to the genre? Does the phraseology match that used in original target-language texts on the same subject? (Sub-language)
  - Are all the word combinations idiomatic? Does the translator observe the rhetorical preferences of the target language? (Idiom)
  - Have the rules of grammar, spelling, punctuation, house style and correct usage been observed? (Mechanics)

- Formal presentation
  - Are there any problems in the way the text is arranged on the page: spacing, indentation, margins? (Layout)
  - Are there any problems of text formatting: bolding, underlining, font type, font size? (Typography)
  - Are there any problems in the way the document as a whole is organized: page numbering, headers, footnotes, table of content? (Organization)

For further information on revision see Brian Mossop's excellent book *Editing and Revising for Translators*, on which this sub-section draws.

Task 13. Avoiding errors

The Health Science Writing Centre at the University of Toronto offers a hit parade of errors in style, grammar, and punctuation in health science writing.

1) Match the error types in column A with the examples in column B (from Bain 2005 at http://www.hswriting.ca/handouts/hitparade.asp). You will find a key at the end of this chapter.
2) Translate the examples into your mother tongue avoiding the errors.

A) Types of error		B) Bain's examples	
1	Lack of agreement: between subjects and verbs, between nouns and pronouns, and between pronouns.	a	It is through this essay that the proposed benefits of active exercise for Chronic Lower Back Pain (CLBP) will be examined.
2	Sentence fragments: a sentence consists of an independent unit with at least a subject and a verb properly connected.	b	A definition that can be employed usefully, according to LaPlante et al. (1993), states that "assistive technology..."
3	Overly-long sentences: a sentence should express only one idea or a clearly connected set of ideas.	c	The council advises physicians at regular intervals to administer the drug.
4	Overuse of passive voice: prefer active verbs to passive verbs, and prefer persons over abstract ideas for the subjects of these verbs.	d	Like a bolt from the blue the idea grabbed him, and it soon took its place as one of his hobby-horses.
5	Faulty parallelism: building parallel elements into a sentence adds clarity and emphasis.	e	Recent discoveries about the weather reveals that several cycles are involved.

6	Vague pronouns: make sure that pronouns such as "it" and "this" refer to something specific.	f	Home care has been expanding tremendously over the past few years partly due to recent technological advances that enable assessments and treatments to be a part of the home setting which at one time could only be performed within the hospital environment.
7	Dangling modifiers: make sure that a modifying phrase or clause has something to modify.	g	The liquid was poured into a glass beaker. Being a strong acid.
8	Squinting modifiers: make sure the modifier clearly refers to the element you want to modify.	h	Much of the literature advocates stretching preparatory to exercise, however, the mechanisms are not well understood.
9	Mixed or dead metaphors: recognize the literal meanings of your metaphors; avoid clichés.	i	In the report it suggests that moderate exercise is better than no exercise at all.
10	Faulty word choice: don't use "fancy" words for their own sake; use a dictionary to check words whose meaning you are not sure of.	j	Eating huge meals, snacking between meals, and too little exercise can lead to obesity.
11	Don't spin empty words; use the minimum number of words.	k	By manipulating the lower back, the pain was greatly eased.
12	Comma splices: use semicolon as well as a conjunctive adverb to join two independent clauses.	l	Explaining the rationale for a treatment can help distil patients' fears.

4.6 Genre shift: Drafting heterofunctional translations

Imagine the following assignment. Your client asks you to translate an original article published in English in the *British Medical Journal* <http://www.bmj. com> into a summary for patients in your mother tongue following the norms of structure, type of information, tenor and length of the summaries for patients published by *Annals of Internal Medicine* at <http://www.annal.com>. Before you go to the next paragraph, have a look at a real example on the web. It will only take you five minutes.

We call this type of assignment genre shift. Genre shifts are performed within the same language (return to chapter 2 to see how, for example, summaries of product characteristics are transformed into patient information leaflets) or between two different languages. In this section, we will focus on the latter. You may also come across expressions such as heterofunctional translation (translation in which the function of the target text is not the same as that of the source text) or transgeneric translation (moving from one genre into another in the process of translation). They all mean the same thing.

In the assignment proposed at the beginning of this section, the source text becomes simply the source of factual information. Communicative purpose, reader's profile, length, structure, tenor, terminological approach, and other key aspects of the target text no longer depend on the source text but rather on the target genre.

A medical text is usually defined as a text written by a specialist for a specialist. However, this apparently straightforward definition does not reflect reality. The text or its translation may not be for another specialist and, what's more, depending on the assignment, the function of the target text can differ from that of the source text. In professional practice, the same specialized text could be translated for different reasons and purposes: as a newspaper report, an internal document, as a synthetic translation, as a sight translation, as an article in a mainstream magazine, or it could be rewritten as a resource text for a TV documentary or radio programme.

Genre shifts as part of the translation process normally occur from more to less specialized genres, and not the other way around. In other words, the target text is normally addressed to less specialized readers, often patients and the general public. Therefore, synthesis of information, terminological simplification (and even determinologization: see chapter 7), paraphrasing and common sense explanations of difficult concepts, and personalization of the language are some of the main procedures we have to use in order to carry out shifts of genre.

A methodology for assignments in which a genre shift is required

1. Define the assignment carefully and in full detail to determine the target genre and the target situation in which the text will be used. At this stage, it is useful to ask oneself 'who will read it and why?', consult web-based documents and other resources, and consider information types and language use. It is also helpful to skim the source text just to have a rough idea of the specific subject matter.

2. Find examples of the target genre in the target language. This will reveal the conventions of the genre that will have to be followed in the drafting of the target text: length, structure, types of information in each part, terminological approach, tenor, style of presentation and so on.
3. Read the source text for information.
4. Select the information that should be transferred to the target genre.
5. Start drafting the target text: (a) Focus on structure. (b) Continue the drafting process following the methodology suggested in this chapter: crafting and improving (see previous sections).

When translating research genres into genres for patients and the general public, the following procedures are frequently used:

- If necessary, expanding relevant information for the target reader. This is designed to reduce complexity by making key meanings explicit
- Shifting from author and content to reader's comprehension
- Adjusting tenor to achieve more personalized communication
- Simplifying structure
- Simplifying syntax
- Determinologizing complex terms
- Using verbs instead of complicated nouns or noun phrases.

Apart from the professional importance of genre shifts in the process of translation, there are two further reasons to take them on board and master them. First, they open up new job opportunities as a medical writer. Second, they improve your abilities as a medical translator in all kinds of assignments, even if there is no genre shift.

4.7 Drafting research papers in English

There is a growing need for researchers all over the world to publish their findings in international journals. Since English has become the *lingua franca* of research communication, translating papers into English – as well as rewriting, revising and editing them – in order to get them published in international biomedical research journals such as *New England Journal of Medicine, The Lancet, British Medical Journal* or *Annals of Internal Medicine* among thousands of others, is now an important market niche for medical translators. In this section we address a key issue: making the text acceptable for publication in an international journal. The editor will require you to observe:

- The Vancouver norms (see chapter 6). These norms are used by all international biomedical research journals.

- The in-house journal's norms. Besides the Vancouver norms, which establish general principles, each particular journal has its own norms.
- Specific guidelines. In order to improve written communication of research, guidelines have been written for a variety of studies such as randomized controlled trials, systematic reviews, economic evaluations, and studies that report on texts of diagnostic methods.
- The main features of research English.

Main features of research English

The Vancouver norms, the in-house requirements of each journal, and specific guidelines are explicit, prescriptive norms. But there are other types of norms that are less visible though equally useful to us. According to Swales and Feak (2004: 16), American academic English, in comparison to other research languages, has been said to:

- Be more explicit about its structure and purposes
- Be less tolerant of asides and digressions
- Use fairly short sentences with less complicated grammar
- Have stricter conventions for subsections and their titles
- Be more loaded with citations
- Rely more on recent citations
- Have longer paragraphs
- Point more explicitly to "gaps" or "weakness" in the previous research
- Use more sentence connectors (words like *however*)
- Place the responsibility for clarity and understanding on the writer rather than the reader.

Your responsability as a translator includes taking this knowledge into account. The tendencies listed above – and others pertinent to other languages or varieties of the same language – should inform your decisions.

4.8 Further tasks

Task 14. Dealing with faulty source texts

Original texts may be faulty in some respects and we may need to improve on them in order to achieve the quality required in the target text. Explain what improvements on the original have been made in the following examples and why.

Example:
Original: We examined eight cases who presented between 1985 and 1993 with

hepatitis.
Gloss: We examined eight patients who presented between 1985 and 1993 with hepatitis.
Explanation: The patient is not a case; a case is an instance of a disease.

Original: Two patients were diagnosed with adenoid cystic carcinoma of the paranasal sinuses.
Gloss: Adenoid cystic carcinoma of the paranasal sinuses was diagnosed in two patients.
Explanation:

Original: Postoperatively, the patient was administered indomethacin at a dose of 100 mg once daily for a month.
Gloss: Postoperatively, indomethacin was administered to the patient at a dose of 100 mg once daily for a month.
Explanation:

Original: During follow up, 25 of 42 patients developed hepatocellular carcinoma.
Gloss: During follow up, hepatocellular carcinoma developed in 25 of 42 patients.
Explanation:

4.9 Further reading

Björk, L., M. Knight and E. Wikborg (1988/1992) *The Writing Process. Composition Writing for University Students*, Lund: Studentlitteratur.

Candlin, C.N. and K. Hyland (eds) (1999) *Writing: Texts, Processes and Practices*, London and New York: Longman.

García, Isabel (ed.) (2005) *El género textual y la traducción. Reflexiones teóricas y aplicaciones pedagógicas*, Bern: Peter Lang.

Hall, G.M. (ed.) (2003) *How to Write a Paper*, London: British Medical Journal Books.

Hedge, Tricia (2005) *Writing*, Oxford: Oxford University Press.

Huth, E.J. (1999) *Writing and Publishing in Medicine*, Baltimore: Williams & Wilkins.

Matthews, J.R., J.M. Bowen and R.W. Matthews (1996/2000) *Successful Scientific Writing. A Step-by-Step Guide for the Biological and Medical Sciences*, Cambridge: Cambridge University Press.

Mossop, Brian (2001) *Revising and Editing for Translators*, Manchester: St. Jerome.

Paradis, J.G. and M.L. Zimmerman (1997) *The MIT Guide to Science and Engineering Communication*, Cambridge and London: The MIT Press.

Swales, J.M. and C.B. Feak (2004) *Academic Writing for Graduate Students. Essential Tasks and Skills*, Michigan: The University of Michigan Press.

------ (2000) *English in Today's Research World. A Writing Guide*, Michigan: The University of Michigan Press.

Key to task 13

1/e; 2/g; 3/f; 4/a; 5/j; 6/i; 7/k; 8/c; 9/d; 10/l; 11/b; 12/h.

---

5. Detecting and solving translation problems

> The strategic competence of translators may be gauged by measuring their awareness of problems and by measuring their ability to achieve communication goals by compensating for losses in translation
>
> Maria Piotrowska (1998: 209)

Overview of chapter

The ability to spot and solve translation problems is at the core of a professional translator's practice (5.1). Translation styles and assignments will determine how close the final text should be to the source text (5.2). Some of the most challenging problems to be solved are ambiguity (5.3), metaphors (5.4) and the expression of cultural perceptions (5.5). As the latter also colour medical texts, an operative definition of culture is suggested here. In the same line, as translations should adapt to the cultural conventions of the target community, both in format and content, appropriate translation procedures are explored. Then, we present a technique to help you improve your decision skills by verbalizing the problem-solving process you follow, so that you can explain your choices to your client in a professional way: Written Protocols (5.6). All this is directly related to the exploratory list of potential medical translation problems, strategies, procedures and solutions which you will find in Appendix 1. The final translation stage, writing, will be dealt with, albeit briefly (5.7), as this topic has been dealt with extensively in chapter 4. Finally, we have included tasks for you to continue practising (5.8) and references for you to carry out further reading (5.9).

5.1 Describing problems, strategies, procedures and solutions

> To return to the matter of correctness, it would clearly be more fruitful to try to see behind apparent errors and characterize the processes that gave rise to them. Many researchers in translation studies are currently concerned with the importance of the process of translation rather than the product.
>
> Stuart Campbell (1991: 331)

Translating is about thinking clearly and *understanding* a text before relaying it in another language. One of the main setbacks an inexperienced medical translator can come across is not spotting that there is a problem in the text. Frequently, novice translators just do not see that there is a problem where an expert translator would pick it up straight away. Therefore, it is crucial to become aware of the fact that not everything may be as easy as it seems at a first glance and improve your *spotting* or *noticing, deciding* and *self-monitoring* skills.

By *spotting* or *noticing* we mean noting, observing or paying special attention to a particular item, generally as a prerequisite for learning. *Deciding* is inherent to the whole process: to making macro- and micro-decisions, to brainstorming and choosing strategies and procedures, as well as to justifying your decisions. *Justifying* is related mainly to final problem-solving by making an informed choice and depends on the development of appropriate *(self)monitoring* skills. It is highly probable that some of these skills may overlap and that different translators will acquire them following different routes (sequential order) and rates (speed).

A translation *problem* can be defined as a (verbal or nonverbal) segment that can be present either in a text segment (micro level) or in the text as a whole (macro level) and that compels the translator to make a conscious decision to apply a motivated translation strategy, procedure and solution from amongst a range of options. A translation *strategy* links the goals of the translation assignment with the necessary procedures (see below) to attain these goals in a given translation context by means of a group of coordinated decisions: parallel or logical thinking, resourcing, classifying, selecting, playing with words, accessing semantic fields and schemata, looking at procedures lists, scanning published translations etc. Translation *procedures* are a range of specific techniques such as explicitation, foot-notes, calques, cultural adaptations, paraphrasing, substitutions, omissions, additions... to re-express the source text in an acceptable way.

Finally, a professional translator should be able to justify or evaluate the translation *solution* chosen in accordance with the translation context and considering text, genre, discourse, function and assignment (Bastin 2000; González Davies and Scott-Tennent 2005; González Davies *et. al* 2001; Hatim and Mason 1990).

Translation problems may be different for different translators. Translating and learning styles along with the personal and professional background of each translator will determine individual perceptions of translation problems. Hence in this volume reference is always made to *potential* problems. Stuart Campbell describes four translator types depending on the *disposition*, related to proficiency and aptitude, or with attitude, related to psychological traits (see chapter 1). Thus, according to this author, the translator's profile can oscillate between being risk-taking or prudent when tackling a translation, and being perseverant or capitulating when dealing with clients or constraints (Campbell 1991: 339). These interact and produce a certain type of translator. The task that follows has been designed to raise your awareness of your translating and translator styles, to help you become aware of the need for a positive translator's self-concept, to explore translation issues related to both your aptitudes and attitudes and reflect on the components of translation competence.

Task 1. What kind of translator are you?

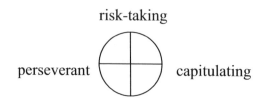

risk-taking

perseverant   capitulating

prudent

Figure 5.1. Translator types (Campbell, 1991)

- Figure 5.1 above represents the four translator types suggested by Campbell.
- Draw a cross at the point where you think the "perfect translator" *should* be.
- Finally, draw another cross where you think you *are*.
- If you are in a group situation, discuss the different places the crosses appear for different translators.

Of course, there is no "right" answer as to the characteristics of a "perfect translator" (perhaps, "in the middle"!): it is the ensuing reflection or discussion with colleagues that matters. In our experience, this usually concerns the positive and negative connotations related to each of the words around the circle (especially, "capitulating", although it is always wise to know when to give in!).

- Finally, try to relate this issue to that of the translator's self-concept and to translation competence: proficiency or aptitude, and attitude (see chapter 1).

Translation problems may arise in any of the three stages involved in translating: reading the source text (see chapters 2 and 3), transferring the text (see this chapter) and writing the target text (see chapter 4). Each of these steps requires complex skills that interact and overlap (see chapter 1). As a revision of what you have seen so far, a section on each stage has been included in this chapter, together with tasks to help consolidate your skills.

5.2 Degrees of fidelity in translation

As mentioned in chapter 1, different translations will require different degrees of fidelity depending on their purpose (*skopos*) and on who will be reading them. A technical text translated for a specialized journal requires a different approach from the translation of a joke, a poem or an advertisment. In the first case, the translation will probably follow the source text very closely using what Hervey et al (1995) call a balanced translation (see below). In the second, the effect on the reader matters more than the actual words or the syntactic layout – the translator will probably opt for an idiomatic or a free translation. To illustrate this point, let's see what happened to the following text written in 1991 to attract business to Barcelona in the year of the Olympic Games (1992) and how the translation procedure has changed after exactly 10 years to adapt to a different readership and also to present-day translation norms in Spain, which are in keeping with the tendency towards recent globalization techniques in advertising. The text appeared as follows in the newspapers:

Source text: *El País* (6.10.1991) – Spanish	Translation: *The European* (4/6.10.1991) English	Source text: *El País* (24.10.2001) – Catalan
Barcelona se escribe con 'B' de Beneficio (literally, "Barcelona is written with a 'B' for Benefit")	Barcelona: it's spelt with 'B' for Business	*business comença amb B* (literally, "business starts with a <u>B</u>" – the underlined letter has been the symbol of the city of Barcelona in recent Town Hall campaigns. Notice the use of the English word in the Catalan sentence.)

There are no changes in the message that has to be conveyed, that is, in *what* has to be said, or in *who* it is addressed to, but there have been changes in *how* it has been rendered for lexical, pragmatic and sociocultural reasons – is this being "unfaithful" to the original text or, on the contrary, has the translator been more faithful by (apparently) moving away from the original words and syntax? It is not usually the most "faithful" in the usual sense of "literal" translation that reads more fluently in the target language as happened, for instance, when Coors' beer "Turn It Loose" slogan was mistranslated into Mexican Spanish as something similar to *Sufra de diarrea* ("Have diarrhea") (www.childrensvaccine.org/files/ – CVP-Materials-Development-Guide-SP.pdf)

The translator, then, has to deal with the following points:

- choosing between keeping mainly the *meaning* or the *effect* of the source text, or both if possible,
- keeping to the translation *assignment*, i.e., writing bearing in mind the purpose of the target text as described by its initiator,
- bearing in mind the *reader* who will receive the message,
- applying appropriate *strategies* and *procedures* to solve potential problems (see Appendix 1),
- *justifying* and *monitoring* the appropriateness of the chosen translation solutions, and
- producing a coherent translation that conforms to the *norms* of the target language and culture as well as to the *text type* required.

Let's take a look at the cline proposed by Hervey et al (1995: 13-14) which helps clarify ideas and answer the question frequently raised in the first training stages: "How close should my translation be to the source text?"

Source language bias   Target language bias

--------------------------------------*------------------*-----------------*-----------------*

  Interlineal   Literal   Faithful   Balanced   Idiomatic   Free

*Figure 5.2. Degrees of fidelity in translation according to ST/TT bias
(Hervey, Higgins and Haywood, 1995)*

Interlineal translation is useful to understand how a language works syntactically, for example, but not to produce fluent texts.

Literal translation moves a step further towards the target language and is "correct" syntactically but can produce calques.

Balanced translation is more fluent and follows the source text closely.

Idiomatic translation tries to convey a similar effect on the reader of the target text.

Free translation emphasizes the effect without changing the message, as has been seen in the example above. It usually involves changing cultural references, dealing with word play and so on, and is sometimes known as **Adaptation**.

   We can conclude along with Hatim and Mason that translation is now mainly considered as "a dynamic process of communication" (1990: 52), *communication* being the key word here, whereas *equivalence*, understood as a one-to-one textual relaying, has no place in translation discussions.

5.3 Improving reading skills: spotting ambiguity

We will start by focusing on reading skills. Novice translators tend to translate without having skimmed the text beforehand. The result is often artificial writing peppered with calques and mistranslations, i.e. an inadequate rendering of the source text for they have not grasped the logic and the message underlying the text as a whole.

One of the trickiest things to detect in a text is ambiguity. The following task aims at raising your awareness by spotting, describing and solving textual comprehension problems related to ambiguity and learning to justify editing choices to improve writing skills, as well as developing logical thinking:

Task 2. Reading skills: Tackling ambiguity

Please contact Maria Gonzalez Davies at <MariaGD@blanquerna.url.edu> to send it to you in a digital format.

5.4 Translating metaphors

Metaphors are also very common in medical texts, in which abstraction and fuzziness can be present (see *Exploring metaphors* in 3.3 Developing text comprehension strategies). Despite aiming for an objective language to explain medical processes, free from what some consider to be obscure references, metaphors, idioms and, sometimes, even proverbs can be found in many scientific texts. Research points to the fact that metaphorical thinking is inborn and makes it easier for us to interpret and filter the messages around us (Lakoff and Johnson 1980, 1999; Brown 2003). Moreover, metaphors in a given field bring to the surface its underlying conceptual system while helping the reader to visualise and understand its construction, its development and its way of facing challenges.

The differentiation between denotative and connotative meaning can be a good starting point for exploring the question of medical metaphors. Denotation refers to the basic meaning of a word, e.g. *rose* (a flower), whereas connotation refers to the emotional associations the same word may carry for different users in different contexts, e.g. *a trip to the seaside will put the roses back in your cheeks.* The challenge in translation comes when the translator has to determine whether the denotative and connotative meaning of a word is the same for the source and target communities or, if only partial or no equivalence can be established, whether the application of a given translation procedure is called for (see below). Different degrees of correspondence can be established:

1. Complete correspondence (same meaning)
Saint Vitus dance (Sydenham's chorea)
Baile de San Vito (corea)
2. Partial correspondence (same meaning, but different lexical or syntactic construction):
I believe it is the greatest intellectual moment in history. Bar none.
Source: Ridley, Matt. (2000) 'Life's twisted plotline', *Time*, Feb 28; 155(8): 80.
Creo que es el descubrimiento intelectual más importante de la historia, sin excepción.
3. Partial correspondence: metaphors, idioms and cultural references (same meaning, different cultural references)
…the medical naysayers got high-cholesterol egg on their faces.
Source: Bjerklie, David (2004) 'Stroke Of Luck. Researchers are finding new ways to deliver treatment when it counts most', *Time*, Feb 16; 163(7): 84.
… los aguafiestas médicos recibieron en la cara una lluvia de huevos con un alto grado de colesterol (the saying is not exactly the same in Spanish, but can be adapted keeping the reference to eggs and high cholesterol by applying sideways chunking (see below).
4. Partial correspondence (polysemy: not all the meanings of the expression can be translated)
Stroke of Luck (Bjerklie 2004: 84) (Stroke: something that happens unexpectedly; also, sudden illness that can cause partial paralysis)
Golpe de suerte (the expression exists in Spanish, but the illness is *apoplejía*, although other possibilities exist)
5. False friends
Lexical or phonetic correspondence, but a different meaning
aerobic
aerobio (not *aeróbico* (aerobiotic))
6. No correspondence
Mr. (appropriate form of address for surgeons in Great Britain)

Common metaphors and idioms in medicine can be related to war, sports, colours, spring, youth, animals, computers, food, or hunting, among other concepts. On the other hand, medicine also influences everyday language that has drawn from the field to illustrate different experiences (although they may not always be accurate, as when emotions are placed in the heart!). Here follow some examples, in alphabetical order:

- baby blues
- blue baby
- catch your death
- coffee grounds (hematemesis or vomiting of blood)
- cohort study (from the divisions of the Roman legions)
- scarlet fever
- Spanish flu
- sugar-coated pill
- swallow a bitter pill
- test battery
- the sugar coating
- to be out cold

- cold sweat
- cold-blooded
- computer virus
- French pox (syphilis)
- German measles
- green medicine
- in cold blood
- invasive procedure
- killer cells

- to feel in heaven
- to feel in hell
- the genome is a book
- white fingers (Raynaud's disease)
- yellow fever / black vomit / the American Plague
- your blood runs cold
- your computer falls sick
- your computer is infected

Task 3. Translating metaphors and idioms in a text

Translate a medical text with metaphors and idioms (see texts A and B, below). Remember and apply the cline of degrees of fidelity and different translation procedures to solve translation problems related to this issue (see 5.2 and Appendix 1).

Text A (*The Economist* 1999: 66)

Asthma

Not to be sneezed at

[…] The lives of both asthma and allergic-rhinitis sufferers could be improved enormously by reliable forecasting of the levels of these pollutants. It would mean, for example, that sufferers could arrange to stay indoors as much as possible on bad days. But although pollen and pollution forecasts are made at the moment, they are usually fairly crude – with countries being divided into a few, large regions.

[…] The Zambon project which is being developed in collaboration with the EU is called, perhaps inevitably, ASTHMA (Advanced System of Teledetection for Healthcare Management of Asthma).

[…] At present, the EAN/EPIS relies on an army of technicians who use microscopes to examine samples taken from air-filters, and identify and count the pollen grains by eye. This can take up to three hours for each slide. The ASTHMA scientists, who are led by Alfredo Ardia, one of Zambon's senior researchers, plan to replace the technician foot-soldiers with a semi-automatic system of pollen recognition based on neural networks.

Text B (*The European* 17-23 June 1999)

Europe in grip of corruption plague
by Roman Rollnick

> The plague of institutionalised corruption and bribery is spreading its cold tentacles across the western democracies of Europe to an unprecedented degree, experts believe.
>
> Italy, […], has finally confronted the contagion and is stamping it out. But cases uncovered in Spain, Britain, Germany, Sweden and France have shown that the local disease may be turning into an epidemic.
> […]
> "We have had a revolution without beheadings, but a political class has been decapitated and tacit support for corruption rejected."
> It is that support which has allowed the plague to spread so widely, experts feel. 'The disease is spreading in countries which regard themselves as firmly established democracies,' said Council secretary-general Peter Leuprecht. 'It is also spreading in the new democracies of eastern and central Europe'.
> Hans Nilsson, a former Swedish judge, agrees that the battle must be fought: 'It is not a question of which countries are the most corrupt; it is simply that graft is human. It is a moral gangrene that will take years and years to fight'.

5.5 Transferring cultural references

> He who does not understand a look, cannot understand long explanations.
>
> (Arab proverb)

As we have already seen, some of the most specialized textual genres, such as research papers and in particular original articles, are highly standardized internationally (see chapter 2). However, as we move along the continuum of medical written communication, genres and texts become more localized in specific cultural settings and, as a consequence, may reflect cultural elements such as:

- Systems of weights and measures
- References to health systems / administrative systems
- Social norms when dealing with ethnic groups, disabled groups, sex groups, etc.
- Varying degrees of formality, tenor...
- Elements of popular knowledge (popular beliefs...)
- Degree of democratization of medical knowledge
- Differences in the relationship patient-physician
- Average medical education of population
- Status and prestige of a given medical tradition

- Differences in basic notions to do with senses, such as hot, cold, sweet, etc.

Here, we will reflect on how culture permeates the texts in each linguistic community determining and shaping style, meanings and terminology, thus becoming a focal point of study and observation for any medical translator.

Defining culture in translation

Despite the many attempts to define culture, no agreement has been reached as to its nature, perhaps unsurprisingly, since instability is its main feature. At first glance, spotting a cultural reference in a text may seem a straightforward task but culture, understood as a manifestation of reality in a given context, is not objective, for its connotations may vary according to beliefs and values, producing different mind maps of the world.

According to David Katan, culture is the framework that helps the individual be a part of a given community; it is a system for orienting experience and forming a mental map of the community (1999: 86).

Basil Hatim, on the other hand, places cultural references on a cline between sociocultural objects with which the social life of given linguistic communities are normally identified, and sociotextual practices, which are influenced by the former (1997: 223).

We would like to suggest the following operative definition of cultural reference adapted to translation purposes (González Davies and Scott-Tennent 2005: 166):

> Any kind of expression (textual, verbal, non-verbal or audiovisual) denoting any material, ecological, social, religious, linguistic or emotional manifestation that can be attributed to a particular community (geographic, socio-economic, professional, linguistic, religious, bilingual, etc.) and would be admitted as a trait of that community by those who consider themselves to be members of it. Such an expression may, on occasions, create a comprehension or a translation problem.

As can be inferred from this definition, one person can belong to several different cultural communities and, although not all the members of the community will accept these manifestations as true or even like them(!), they will recognize them as belonging to their community.

Noticing cultural references: translation procedures I

Observing and reading about the communities involved can be accompanied by the exploration and practice of techniques that can help to solve the translation problems further such as chunking, proposed by Katan (1999: 148-157), i.e. finding alternatives to the cultural blocking problem. Through chunking up, down or sideways, the translator changes the size and the viewpoint of the problematic segment when there is no correspondence: from subatomic to universal, from concrete to abstract, from one way of viewing the world to another, from one cultural framework to another.

Here are examples of each, with reference to translation into Spanish. Think about the translation into your own target language.

Chunking up: a specific (subatomic) segment becomes general (universal). The key question to ask is 'What is this an example of?' (search for an hyperonym)
Example
'Mark the spot where they stopped by placing a bean bag or a piece of tape on the floor.'
(Source: ATS Statement: Guidelines for the Six-Minute Walk Test", The Official Statement of the American Thoracic Society, (2002). *American Journal Critical Care Med*, 166: 111-117).
Bean bag: a large free-form bag or cushion filled with beads of polystyrene.
Possible translation into Spanish: *cojín* (cushion).

Chunking down: moving from a universal term to a subatomic one. The question to ask is 'What is a specific example of this?' (search for a hyponym)
Example
'Like any other NHS medical treatment, the art classes will be free [...] Patients with mental health problems are to be prescribed painting, sculpting and creative writing on the NHS, instead of drugs.'
(Source: Walton, Richard and Mark Bartram (2000) *Initiative.* Cambridge: Cambridge University Press, 115).
In Spanish, 'Art classes' could become *clases de pintura, escultura o escritura creativa*, for *clases de arte* refers only to painting and would not be appropriate in this context.

Chunking sideways: Finding a reference with similar characteristics. 'What is another example of this?'
Example
'Clearing snow off your car'
(Source: E.F. Juniper, G.H.Guyatt, R.S. Epstein, P.J. Ferrie, R. Jaeschke and T.K. Hiller (1992). 'Evaluation of impairment of health related quality of life in asthma: development of a questionnaire for use in clinical trials', *Thorax*, Feb, 47(2): 76-83.)
As there is not as much snow in Spain as in Canada, a similar activity has to be chosen.

Possible translation: *Lavar el coche* [Wash your car].

Task 4. Adapting a questionnaire for use in clinical trials.

Below you will find part of the article E.F. Juniper, G.H.Guyatt, R.S. Epstein, P.J. Ferrie, R. Jaeschke and T.K. Hiller (1992). 'Evaluation of impairment of health related quality of life in asthma: development of a questionnaire for use in clinical trials', *Thorax*, Feb, 47(2): 76-83, which we have transcribed here. Translate it into your target language for a lung specialist in a country that is not Canada where some of the 'Canadian' activities may not be carried out usually by a large part of the population.

***

Appendix: Asthma quality of life questionnaire (interviewer)

The questionnaire includes 32 questions. Each has one of four sets of seven response options, identified by the colour of the card (...) First subjects are asked to identify activities in which they are limited by their asthma. If more than five activities are identified, they are asked to choose the five most important. To ensure that all possible relevant items are considered, subjects are presented with the following prompts:

- Bicycling
- Clearing snow off your car*
- Dancing
- Doing home maintenance
- Doing housework
- Gardening*
- Hurrying
- Jogging, exercising or running
- Laughing
- Mopping or scrubbing the floor
- Mowing the lawn
- Playing with pets
- Playing with children
- Playing sports
- Shovelling snow*
- Singing
- Doing regular social activities
- Having sexual intercourse
- Talking

- Running upstairs or uphill
- Vacuuming
- Visiting friends or relatives
[...]
    * Included only in studies conducted in the appropriate season

***

As you may have noticed, some elements in the source questionnaire must be adapted so that the target questionnaire is valid for the target culture you have chosen. You will have to think of activities that require a similar degree of exertion and apply some of the translation procedures we have seen above. For example, in Spain the following are not usual:

- Gardening
- Mowing the lawn
- Shovelling snow
- Vacuuming
- Woodwork or carpentry

Cultural elements in medical communication: translation procedures II

Although culture permeates texts and can be considered at a macro-level, affecting genres, conventions, functions, styles and tone, and so on (see below), specific translation procedures for solving micro-level translation problems related to cultural references such as those proposed by Hervey, Higgins and Haywood's cline (1995: 20) can prove useful:

SL bias   TL bias
------------------------------------*------------------*------------------*------------------*

Exoticism   Cultural   Calque   Transliteration   Communicative   Cultural
            borrowing   translation   transplantation

Figure 5.3. Translation procedures and SL/TL bias (Hervey, Higgins and Haywood, 1995)

Here follows a brief explanation for each of the procedures. As a starting point for reflection, an example will be given in English-Spanish, for this is a language combination with which we usually work and which we teach. Try to find similar examples in your own language combination when translating. Whether, as translators, we will choose those procedures closer to the target language and culture or those that will keep the source language and culture "flavour" of the text will depend on the translation assignment (e.g. if we are asked to localize the text, we will have to adapt it to the target culture and probably use cultural transplantation instead of exoticisms and so on).

Exoticism: The source language is kept with no changes in the translation: e.g. *rash* in Spanish (not accepted in the prescriptive reference dictionary of the *Real Academia de la Lengua Española* (RAE) www.rae.es, although this word is widely used by medical practitioners in Spain).

Cultural Borrowing: the source language word or expression is rendered without change in the target language (but, in the Spanish case, has been accepted by the RAE), e.g. *lifting* (face lift or lifting) instead of *estiramiento facial*.

Calque: the target language is similar to the source language word or expression but does not conform to target language rules, although it may be widely used e.g. *linfoma no Hodgkin* (non-Hodgkin lymphoma NHL).

Transliteration: the cultural referent is changed according to the phonic or graphic conventions of the target language, e.g. scanner is *escáner*.

Communicative: the source language referent has an identifiable correspondence in the target language that is not a literal translation, e.g. foot-and-mouth disease is *fiebre aftosa* or *glosopeda* in Spanish.

Cultural transplantation: the reference has been completely adapted to the target culture, has been substituted by a reference which is more in accordance with its norms or has been changed for ideological reasons, e.g. Spanish tourniquet is *garrote*.

Task 5. Translate by adapting language to culture

This activity will help you to translate considering not only the linguistic, but also the cultural features of texts as well as adapting them to different community viewpoints and to different ways of conveying similar information.

First, analyze the linguistic and cultural features of Patient Information Leaflets for the same or a similar medical product, but issued in different countries (see sample below). Ideally, you should do this with colleagues from different language and cultural backgrounds. Parallel texts can be found on the Internet (see chapter 2 for urls), and some leaflets are written in different languages.

Once you have spotted or discussed possible similarities and differences, start translating using a localizing strategy (see above). Have you managed to convey the cultural features? How does language convey culture?

Sample texts (British English / European Spanish)

Boots Foam Protective Bandage
Before application, ensure that the area to be treated is clean and dry. Then, with sharp scissors cut the length of Boots Foam Protective Bandage that is required and place over the painful area. Boots Foam Protective Bandage can be cut at any angle and if applied to a finger, can be cut with a 'nick' in the side...

Apósitos plásticos callicidas Salve
Lavar el pie con agua caliente y secarlo cuidadosamente.
Aplicar Callicida Salve directamente sobre el callo o zona afectada y dejar actuar sin retirarlo 3 días.
Levantar el apósito y lavar el pie con agua caliente.
[...]

Communicating medical information to patients and what the experts say: bridging cultural gaps

'Emotion' is also a key word in the operative definition of culture suggested above. It is undeniable that it plays a central role in the relationship between doctors and patients as well as between writers/translators and readers, especially when they belong to different communities. An increasing number of publications and courses that deal with this issue are underway, such as that developed by the UCI (University of California, Irvine) to 'prepare future doctors to serve a growing Latino population that often lacks access to health care'. It offers both 'intensive language and cultural training', for the organizers believe 'doctors should not only know how to heal but also understand the culture and lifestyle of their patients, including diet, problems in their neighborhoods, and family ties' (Perkes 2003). It is extremely useful to be aware of these issues and to complement your readings with texts on community interpreting, where transcultural misunderstandings are also discussed because:

> The community interpreter has a very different role and responsibilities from a commercial or conference interpreter. She is responsible for enabling professional and client, with very different backgrounds and perceptions and in an unequal relationship of power and knowledge, to communicate to their mutual satisfaction. (Shackman 1984, in Bowen 2000: 234)

Margareta Bowen (2000: 234) goes on to explain the circumstances surrounding community interpreters and their clients, which are also pertinent and can be adapted to doctor-patient communication situations around the world whenever two communities are involved:

> Even if they have been living in their host country for years, their community, like New York's "Little Italy" or the Polish area of Chicago, has protected them from the need to learn English until they need social security or health care. The settings are hospitals and doctors' offices, schools, the various offices dealing with immigrant matters, housing and social security, and police stations. [...] the language level may be quite different from that of a diplomatic conference: regional variations and dialects can be a problem. [...] The clients are worried, afraid, and sometimes illiterate. They find themselves in strange surroundings. Add to these difficulties the fact that the professionals – the doctors, nurses, police officers, social workers etc. – are usually in a hurry. [...] In a nutshell, community interpreters need people skills as well as language and cultural knowledge – and interpreting know-how.

Moreover, research is being carried out on cross-cultural communication that can be found in specialized medical journals with articles such as: 'Vamos a Traducir los MRV (let's translate the VRM): linguistic and cultural inferences drawn from translating a verbal coding system from English into Spanish' by Caro and Stiles (*Psychiatry* 1997: 233-247), 'Using cross-cultural input to adapt the Functional Assessment of Chronic Illness Therapy (FACIT) scales' by Lent et al (*Acta Oncologica* 1999: 695-702), or 'Cuestionario de calidad de vida en pacientes con asma: la versión española del Asthma Quality of Life Assessment' by Sanjuás et al (*Archivos de Bronconeumología* 1995: 219-226). All this research is related to translation protocols and on how a given translation bias can influence the interpretation and discussion of results in medical research, especially when direct communication with the patients is involved. Cultural misunderstandings may arise from subtle signs such as non-verbal language, politeness strategies such as turn-taking, speech or text rhythm, degrees of formality, and so on.

Can the problems in textual translation and personal communication be solved in any way, albeit approximately? There are strategies and procedures published in works in Translation Studies and in Linguistics and Pragmatics, that we can cover briefly here to give a general outline of possible paths to learn to establish a distance between the source language and the target language cultural frameworks, and operate according to motivated choices that aim at reconciling both (see above).

In this vein, Speech Act Theory is a relevant area for translators to explore (Austin 1962, Searle 1969). This theory studies and analyzes what people do when they speak. Their meaning can be literal or locutive (e.g. "I've got a headache"), intentional or illocutive ("I've got a headache" *really* means "Could you bring me an aspirin, please?"), or perlocutive, i.e. creating an effect on the listener (e.g. you have to bring me the aspirin because my tone indicates I'm your boss).

Likewise, Grice's Conversational Maxims (1975) present the rules that can be followed or broken in conversation:

- **quantity**: as much information as is needed should be given, not more and not less;
- **quality**: the truth should be told, not anything for which there is no evidence;
- **relevance**: say only what matters;
- **manner**: be clear, direct and avoid ambiguity.

Cooperation and sincerity are, supposedly, at the root of the conversational exchange, but the maxims can be broken forcing the listener to read between lines, as it were, and detect the **implicatures**, i.e. what has not been openly stated.

Conflicts may arise when two communities use Speech Acts or Grice's Maxims in different ways, so it follows that translators and interpreters should be familiar with both viewpoints to overcome possible divergences. Katan (1999: 178-181), following Hall's contexting principle (1983: 61), suggests that communities are biased towards being either HCC (high context communities) if communication takes place through context rather than through texts, or LCC (low context communities) if the contrary takes place. HCC communities are tightly woven and base their communication and decisions on relationships, indirectness, flexibility in meaning, social and personal appearance, and circumstances. They favour indirect speech acts and dense, elaborate texts. LCC, on the other hand, are more loosely knit and communicate and decide depending on facts, direct speech acts, consistency, substance, and rules. He goes on to present Victor's (1992: 143) cline of a context ranking of cultures:

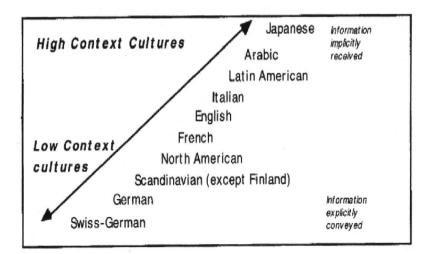

Figure 5.4. Context ranking of cultures (Victor, 1992 in Katan, 1999)

This cline is based on geographical differences but, as has been mentioned above, this is not the only possible community division. However, these suggestions may serve as tentative guidelines, and be taken as useful starting points for conscious-ness-raising, reflection and discussions concerning cultural diversity, but not as deterministic and unmovable claims on cultural stereotypes.

Task 6. Degrees of cultural immersion.

How many foreign languages do you speak? How many communities do you think you belong to? How many countries have you visited? Try and relate Hanvey's classification of degrees of cultural immersion (1992: 182-192), which we reproduce below, to your own experience. According to this author, there are four levels of cultural immersion:

Level 1: **Facts, Stereotypes and Deficiencies**. At this stage there is still a large comprehension gap between the source culture and the target culture.

Level 2: **Shallow comprehension**. Subtle traits in the thought and behav-iour of the foreign culture community are discerned.

Level 3: **In-Depth Comprehension**. The target culture is accepted and the reasons behind certain modes of behaviour, understood.

Level 4: **Empathy**. This stage can only be achieved by immersion in the foreign culture.

Sophisticated cross-cultural communication almost certainly requires translators to be at stages three or four. This is definitely one of the most fascinating areas in which a translator can be immersed, complex and rewarding as well as difficult to master.

Can we apply this to medical translation or interpreting? Have you ever visited a doctor abroad or had to address him or her in a foreign language? Reflect on your experience.

Task 7. Explaining illness in different cultures

A possible follow-up to the previous activity, especially if you have the opportunity of working with colleagues from other cultures, could be to explain different common complaints from different points of view:

- Which home remedies are used in different communities?
- How are the complaints explained to children, for example?
- What happens with more serious diseases?
- Are there any taboo diseases?

5.6 Transference skills: Written Protocols (WP)

Professional translators should not only translate well, but should also be able to justify their translation choices to a client, if required to do so. They use a wide range of strategies and procedures to solve translation problems, always bearing in mind that a medical translation should keep the message and effect of the source text, but adapt them if required by the assignment or the purpose of the target text.

The written protocol (WP) which we describe below has been designed to help you make visible your translating and reasoning processes: to develop problem spotting and solving skills, to become aware of translation problems in a text and to reflect on the process of translation and justify your choices in a professional way (see 5.1).

These protocols have proved to be effective in improving our medical translation students' awareness of their thinking process and of their evolution in the acquisition of translation competence. In different studies (González Davies et al, 2001; González Davies and Scott-Tennent 2005, Scott-Tennent and González Davies, forthcoming), it was observed that problems may vary from student to student according mainly to their aptitudes and background knowledge.

One of the main aims of WP, is to build up a personal inventory of translation strategies and procedures (see Appendix 1), depending on individual aptitudes and attitudes, thus encouraging reflective learning. In a classroom setting, they also encourage reflective teaching by helping the teacher follow the students' evolution and have a closer understanding of their translation choices

The standard WP sheet consists of three columns (see below): the first should include the problem found in the source text, the second, the range of possible solutions and the strategies used to arrive at them; the third, the final solution and a justification for the choice.

Take a look at an example to see how it works:

- in the first column there is a student's real translation problem when translating an assignment,
- in the second, the steps that have been followed to solve it and the tentative solutions arrived at, and
- in the third, the final solution and its justification.

TRANSLATION PROBLEM	STEPS OR STRATEGIES AND TENTATIVE SOLUTIONS	FINAL SOLUTION AND ITS JUSTIFICATION
- peak flow meters	1) *medidor de flujo espiratorio máximo* 2) *flujómetro* - monolingual dictionaries (English and Spanish); - bilingual paper and online dictionaries: Eurodicautom, Stedman; - Fernando Navarro's *Diccionario de dudas*; - parallel texts (*PubMed*).	*medidor de flujo espiratorio máximo* I have consulted people with asthma and a lung specialist, and searched in the sources cited in the previous column.

Figure 5.5. Sample student's Written Protocol

In Appendix 1, you will find an exploratory list of the most frequent medical translation problems we have come across as well as suggested strategies and procedures that can be used to arrive at appropriate solutions. It is important to note that the list is open to consideration and further additions, that it is not our intention to establish one-to-one correspondences between the listed problems and solutions, and that they are all equally relevant. The chosen strategies, procedures and final solutions will depend on many factors, such as those already mentioned in previous chapters in the book. To emphasize this point, they are in alphabetical order.

In Jack Segura's words, a translator is 'a good researcher and a good reporter' (1999: 9). Internalizing this principle and becoming aware of a wide range of possibilities to produce an appropriate final target text can save years of individual guessing and note-taking!

Task 8. Building a list of translation problems, strategies and solutions

Have a look at Appendix 1. The sources for this list of problems and solutions are several and varied:

- our own experience as translators of medical texts
- classroom observation and discussions
- professional translators' consultations on e-lists such as MedTrad
- academic papers by other medical translators as well as medical translation teachers and translation scholars: Baker 1992, Jammal 1999, Lee-Jahnke 2001, Segura 1999, Wakabayashi 1996 (all references are here instead of embedded in the appendix to smooth the reading process).

The main *concepts* are followed, as needed, by potential *problems* to be solved (*potential* because different translators may have different problems), translation *strategies*: steps to access acceptable procedures, and translation *procedures*: potential final solutions.

The main task suggested here to practise and improve problem spotting and solving skills is to build upon the guidelines in Appendix 1 with your own observations as you carry out your translations with the help of the *Written Protocols* (see above).

Task 9. Translating a text to explore translation problems and solutions

Translate the following text for a similar publication in your target language. First, spot potential problems and think of different solutions for each one, following the *Written Protocols* above. Use the most appropriate translation strategies and procedures included in the list in Appendix 1.

You may apply other strategies and procedures, of course. If you do so, add them to the grid.

***

Tuesday, Feb. 20, 2001

Fated to Be Fat?

A blood test on the horizon could show us who's destined to be dainty – and who needs to keep a sharp eye on the bathroom scale

By Jessica Reaves

Here's a quick quiz:

Which would you rather do:

A) Have somebody prick your finger for a drop of blood
B) Diet constantly in a never-ending quest to lose weight
C) Spend your entire life dealing with food urges and worrying about weight-related health problems.

If you chose A, you may be in luck. According to Rockefeller University researcher Dr. Sarah Leibowitz, we could someday see a simple blood test that would determine a child's risk for obesity – and thus enable appropriate eating behaviors to be instilled at an early age.

Don't get too excited – the test is still years away. But as Dr. Leibowitz announced Monday at the annual meeting of the American Association for the Advancement of Science, the methodology has proven extremely successful in rats, whose appetite and weight gain mechanisms are incredibly similar to those of humans.

The rats in question were fed a low-fat diet until they reached what can best be described as "rodent puberty" – at which point they were all given a very high-fat meal. (Sort of the rat equivalent of freshman year at college). The rats whose blood showed a very high incidence of triglycerides (i.e., fat) after the meal were the same rats who became obese.

Sure, Leibowitz exposed the rats to a veritable wonderland of fattening food, and placed no limits on the rats' consumption – but remember, she was trying to recreate the temptations we humans face every single day. Even given equal access to the unhealthy fare, the rats who were doomed to really expand were far more likely than their slimmer peers to gorge themselves on the fattening foods.

Obese humans, scientists speculate, gain weight because they consume too much fat. Let's say I eat french fries every day with lunch. That fat is tucked away in my body for safekeeping (hello, lovehandles), a survival instinct that leaves my body craving still more fat to perform its normal functions. If we were all living on berries and nuts and only rarely eating meats and fats, nutritionists say, we'd probably use up all of our stored fat between big meals, and we wouldn't have any weight problems. But in our sedentary society, most of us struggle to exercise at all – let alone perform all the hunting and gathering it would take to burn off all the fatty foods tempting us from the supermarket aisles.

If Dr. Leibowitz's test becomes a reality, it would present a novel weapon in the fight against fat – those who are preordained to become obese would be indisputably forewarned. Armed with that knowledge, they could learn how to moderate their diets, stay healthy and recognize the warning signs of serious weight problems. The key to beating obesity, as with most illnesses, is prevention.

After all, as so many of us know, it's a heck of a lot easier to wave aside that second piece of cheesecake in the first place than it is to take it off once it's made itself comfortable along our hips and stomachs.

(Source: J. Reaves, J. (2001). 'Fated to Be Fat?'. *Time*, Tuesday, Feb. 20. Available at: http://www.time.com/time/health/article/0,8599,100023,00. html)

5.7 Facing problems in the production stage: writing

Reading, transferring and writing processes are related and the stages for each one can overlap. Our adaptation of Wright's (1999: 96) performance design can help the visualization of the bridges that are built between the three steps:

1. Identify audience and, in particular, the design needs of subgroups such as specialist or non-specialist readers.
2. Specify the decisions or actions that readers should be able to take using the information.
3. Determine the target text content and structure from an analysis of the full information needs of all the subgroups of users, if necessary dividing the content across sources – e.g. label and leaflet.
4. Prepare a draft translation that meets the design constraints.
5. Performance-test the draft with members of the target audience.
6. Revise the draft in the light of insights gained from performance testing.
7. Performance-test the revision.
8. Iterate stages 6 and 7 until the criteria specified in 2 are met.

The task that follows has been designed to improve your final product by minding the process. Also,

*   to help you acquire appropriate reading habits,

- to understand that reading for translation requires specific skills,
- to understand that you cannot translate until you have understood the text,
- to understand that you have
- to identify the text types before translating,
- to help you spot potential problems and think about means to solve them before translating the text.

In short, it puts into practice the performance steps outlined above. If you carry out this or a similar procedure with each translation, it will become an automatic habit.

Task 10. From reading the source text to writing the target text

First, skim through the whole text below. Design a translation brief. Then, cover the text and pinpoint the text type and purpose both of the source text and of the translation, which will depend on the assignment you have designed for yourself.

Go on to discuss the degree of formality, the possible segments you will have to look up or which may pose problems, possible questions for a potential client, and the parallel texts and reference works you may need.

Once the basic previous background work has been done, go on to the next stage, which consists of paraphrasing the text in your own target language words, as if you were explaining it to someone.

Then, do the same with each sentence. Do not write anything down until you have understood the sentence. At this stage, it is preferable to start writing because you may discover that you have rendered a perfectly acceptable translation orally, but have then forgotten it if you have gone on to the next sentence without writing it down.

Carrying out this task systematically will help you improve your translations, you will not take as much time to do them, and will become more confident about your final rendering, mainly because you will now be writing about something you *understand*. Also, you will not spend so much time as you used to looking words up in the dictionary because you will have unconsciously applied strategies such as remembering the words, guessing them through the context, or exchanging information. Besides, by verbalizing the text, you will gradually improve the coherence and internal structure of your translations.

***

Sleep inspires insight

Insight denotes a mental restructuring that leads to a sudden gain of explicit knowledge allowing qualitatively changed behaviour. Anecdotal reports on scientific discovery suggest that pivotal insights can be gained through sleep. Sleep consolidates recent memories and, concomitantly, could allow insight by changing their representational structure. Here we show a facilitating role of sleep in a process of insight. Subjects performed a cognitive task requiring the learning of stimulus – response sequences, in which they improved gradually by increasing response speed across task blocks. However, they could also improve abruptly after gaining insight into a hidden abstract rule underlying all sequences. Initial training establishing a task representation was followed by 8 h of nocturnal sleep, nocturnal wakefulness, or daytime wakefulness. At subsequent retesting, more than twice as many subjects gained insight into the hidden rule after sleep as after wakefulness, regardless of time of day. Sleep did not enhance insight in the absence of initial training. A characteristic antecedent of sleep-related insight was revealed in a slowing of reaction times across sleep. We conclude that sleep, by restructuring new memory representations, facilitates extraction of explicit knowledge and insightful behaviour.

Source: Wagner U., S. Gais, H. Haider , R. Verleger, and J. Born (2004) 'Sleep inspires insight', *Nature,* Jan 22; 427(6972): 352-5.

5.8 Further tasks

Task 11. Translating advertisements with medical references

When carrying out this activity, you can practise cultural transference (e.g. localizing, or adapting the text to the target culture, and globalizing, or adapting the text to an international audience), analyze the characteristics of different text types and develop your creativity skills.

We suggest that, in the first place, you write a list of the characteristics of advertising language (verbal and visual) (see, for instance, Adab 2001, Corpas Pastor et al 2002, de Pedro 1996, Tatilon 1990).

Look for a couple of advertisements related to a medical topic. See whether the features you had identified appear. Can you identify others?

Translate one of the advertisements and note the problems you encounter using the written protocol.

Task 12. Phraseology: avoiding calques and redundancy

The main aims of this task are to edit sentences with calques, ambiguity or redundancy, to justify the corrections, to rewrite sentences and texts (text editing), and to self monitor final translations.

In the table below, you will find some examples of frequent expressions which can be improved upon in the left-hand column together with a proposal for improvement in the right-hand column:

A considerable amount of	Much
As a consequence of	because
is defined as	is
Of a red colour	red
On a daily basis	daily
It is obvious in fig. 8 that…	(see figure 8)

Now you will find three paragraphs taken from authentic examples of genres which are identified in brackets after each one. Each can be improved upon by rewriting. If you can do this activity with a colleague, you can compare your solutions and try to justify them to each other. Possible solutions are proposed at the end of this chapter.

Paragraph 1

The medical instrument does not need to use fire and you are not worried about scald. […] It can cure such diseases as wind-wetness evil abominal pain… […] The instrument arranges from large, medium and small sizes.
(Plastic Medical Magnetic Jar Manual).

Paragraph 2

We present the cytologic findings of a fine-needle aspiration breast lesion with a typical histology for adenoid cystic carcinoma. The aspirate yielded a very cellular smears with a monomorphic population of small slightly atypical cells […] suspicious for malignancy.
(Abstract)

Paragraph 3

A 75-year-old- cattle farmer presented to the Emergency Room in February 1991 with severe pain, swelling and progressive limitation of motion of the right kenee for the last two weeks [...] The patient persisted afebrile. The negative results so far obtained and the rural environment of the patient raised the suspition of a brucellar infection.
(Case Report).

Task 13. Comparing world visions: Metaphors in medical language

Write a list of 10 metaphors, idioms or proverbs that you find in medical texts. Write the source text reference next to the entries. Then translate the metaphors, idioms and proverbs and make a list of any useful resources you have found.

5.9 Further reading

On translation problems and solutions

Baker, Mona (1992) *In Other Words*, London and New York: Routledge.

Beeby, Allison, Doris Ensinger and Marisa Presas (eds) (2000) *Investigating Translation: Selected papers from the 4th International Congress on Translation, Barcelona, 1998*, Amsterdam and New York: John Benjamins. Especially Section II.

González Davies, Maria (coord) (2003) *Secuencias. Tareas para la enseñanza interactiva de la traducción especializada*, Barcelona: Octaedro.

González Davies, Maria, Christopher Scott-Tennent and Fernanda Rodríguez (2001) 'Training in the Application of Translation Strategies for Undergraduate Scientific Translation Students', *Meta* 46 (4): 737-744.

González Davies, Maria and Eva Espasa (2003) 'Traducción de textos científicos: medicina y medio ambiente', in Maria González Davies (coord.) *Secuencias. Tareas para el aprendizaje interactivo de la traducción especializada*, Barcelona: Octaedro. 39-63.

Kussmaul, Paul (1995) *Training the Translator*, Amsterdam and New York: John Benjamins

Lörscher, W. (1991) *Translation Performance, Translation Process, and Translation Strategies. A Psycholinguistic Investigation*, Tübingen: Narr.

Piotrowska, M. (1998) 'Towards a model of strategies and techniques for teaching translation', in Ann Beylard-Ozeroff, Jana Králová and Barbara Moser-Mercer (eds) *Translators' Strategies and Creativity: Selected Papers from the 9th International Conference on Translation and Interpreting, Prague, September 1995. In honor of Jiří Levý and Anton Popovič*, Amsterdam and Philadelphia: John

Benjamins, 207-211

Scott- Tennent, Christopher and Maria González Davies (forthcoming) 'Effects of Specific Training on the Ability to Deal with Cultural Referents in Translation', *Meta*.

On community interpreting

Angelelli, Claudia V. (2004) *Revisiting the Interpreter's Role: A study of conference, court, and medical interpreters in Canada, Mexico, and the United States*, Amsterdam and Philadelphia: John Benjamins.

Bowen, Margareta (2000) 'Community Interpreting', *AIIC*, September: 234. Also available at: http://www.aiic.net/ViewPage.cfm/page234.htm.

Perkes, Courtney (2003) 'A medical speciality in treating Hispanics – New curriculum at UCI will instruct doctors in culture and language', The Orange County Register: June 11, Hispanicvista.com Inc. [Available at: http://www2.ocregister.com/ocrweb/ocr/article.do?id=43085]

Pöchhacker, Franz and Miriam Shlesinger (eds) (2005) *Healthcare Interpreting: Discourse and Interaction*, Special issue of *Interpreting* 7(2).

Roberts, Roda P., Silvana E. Carr, Diana Abraham and Aideen Dufour (eds) (2000) *The Critical Link 2: Interpreters in the Community: Selected papers from the Second International Conference on Interpreting in legal, health and social service settings, Vancouver, BC, Canada, 19–23 May 1998*, Amsterdam and Philadelphia: John Benjamins.

'What is community interpreting?' at: http://lrc.wfu.edu/community_interpreting/pages/community-interpreting-cont.htm.

On culture

González Davies, Maria and Christopher Scott-Tennent (2005) 'A Problem-Solving and Student-Centred Approach to the Translation of Cultural References', *Meta* 50(1): 160-179 [Monograph *Enseignement de la traduction dans le monde*].

Hanvey, R.G. (1992) 'Culture', in R.C. Scarcella and R.L. Oxford (eds) *The Tapestry of Language Learning. The Individual in the Classroom*, Boston Mass.: Heinle and Heinle, 182-192.

Hervey, Sandor, Ian Higgins and Louise M. Haywood (1995) *Thinking Spanish Translation. A Course in Translation Method: Spanish to English*, London: Routledge. (Also, Arabic, French, German and Italian Translation in the same series)

Katan, David (2004) *Translating cultures. An introduction for translators, interpreters and mediators,* Manchester: St. Jerome. 2nd edition.

Key to Task 11

Paragraph 1
This instrument does not need to be heated, so there is no danger of

---

burning. It is used in treating abdominal pain. The instrument is available in large, medium and small sizes.

Paragraph 2
We present the cytologic findings of a fine-needle aspiration breast lesion with a typical histology for adenoid cystic carcinoma. The aspirate yielded distinct cellular smears with a monomorphic population of small slightly atypical cells, possibly malignant.

Paragraph 3
A 75-year-old- cattle farmer checked into the Emergency Room in February 1991 with severe pain, swelling and progressive limitation of motion of the right knee during the previous two weeks [...] The fever persisted. The negative findings obtained and the rural environment in which the patient lived suggested a brucellar infection.

6. Using resources to solve problems

> Il est primordial d'initier les étudiants à une lecture critique des textes
> parallèles afin qu'ils puissent se documenter de façon efficace.
>
> Hannelore Lee-Jahnke (2001: 151)

Overview of chapter

Before starting to search for information, we will have a look at the whole
picture (6.1). As you gain experience, you will build up your own printed and
digital library according to your particular needs. But some basic resources are
provided here as a starting point (6.2). The Internet has become the main source
of information and help for professional translators; however, it should be used
critically (6.3). Solutions to translation problems are often found in existing texts
(6.4) and by consulting other professionals (6.5). Some tasks (6.6) and suggestions
for further reading (6.7) are presented at the end of the chapter.

6.1 Organizing yourself

We may need to consult all kinds of information sources during the three main
stages of any translation assignment: 1) when reading and trying to understand the
source text (see chapter 3); 2) when drafting and revising the target text (see chapter 4), and 3) in solving translation problems during transfer (see chapter 5).

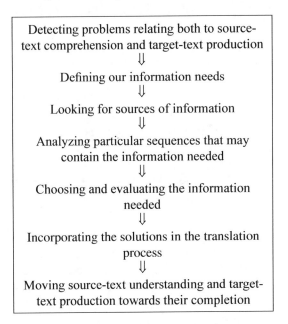

Figure 6.1. Searching and consulting in the translation process

The obstacles that translators regularly come up against fall roughly into two main types: those which hinder a true understanding of the original (see chapter 3) and those which may adversely affect the completion of a reliable finished product which will satisfy the client (see chapters 4 and 5).

All problems boil down to a lack of information of one kind or another. Our needs will determine the types of materials and sources we consult and the type of preparatory research we undertake. It is vital to conduct a careful needs analysis before beginning searches. We need to approach our searches efficiently so as to produce a satisfactory outcome for the minimum of effort. Time, after all, is money, at least in professional practice.

Once we have determined where our problem lies, whether in understanding the original, or completing the target text, it is important to define as precisely as possible just what it is that we need. Here we are dealing with essentially four different types of information.

1) Knowledge of the topic

This is general information that serves as an introduction to one or several areas of knowledge and provides us with a background to the theme of the text. Armed with this information, we can delve deeper into the meaning of the text – particularly important when dealing with a highly specialized topic. Our sources will include, inter alia, encyclopaedias, textbooks, and continuing education articles.

2) Terms and other units of specialized knowledge (usk)

This includes specialized terminology, abbreviations, nomenclatures, symbols, and set phrases. Any usk consists of a concept (content) and a denomination (form). Therefore information about terms and other usks comprises both conceptual and formal information. Scientific and technical concepts may be extremely complex and hard to grasp but expanded definitions of these concepts will often help us to understand, process and finally re-express them in our translation. Indeed, one of the best ways of acquiring conceptual information is by making use of clear, full and reliable definitions of the concepts we have to deal with. Additional useful conceptual aids are images – photos, illustrations, drawings, diagrams, or videos – often easily found on the Internet, which is an excellent source of multi-media materials.

Scientific and technical translation usually requires familiarity with precise terminology in the target language. The more specialized the text, the more the need for this and the greater the time needed for checking to ensure accuracy.

Translators can have recourse to specialized glossaries and dictionaries, but encyclopaedias, textbooks, research papers, experts in the field, and so forth are also valuable sources of information on terminology. Occasionally, we may find that there is no established equivalent term in the target language. In such cases, it is vital to contact other translators and experts in the field in order to find an acceptable rendering.

3) Information on text genre

Difficulties often arise with the conventions governing different genres (see chapter 2), especially when that of the original is not the same as that of the translation. Even if they are the same, there may well be important differences in the two languages, which need to be addressed. These may be structural, discursive, stylistic, terminological, phraseological, and so forth. The best way of familiarizing ourselves with these kinds of conventions is to pay attention to parallel texts in the target language.

4) Linguistic information

This is needed not only to resolve grammatical uncertainties but also to improve the flow and readability of the translation. Linguistic information can be found in dictionaries of false friends, dictionaries of synonyms, thesauruses, grammars, and style manuals.

Types of information needed	Resources
1) Topic	Encyclopaedias, text books, web pages, parallel texts, field experts, and so forth.
2) Terms and other usks	Dictionaries, glossaries, encyclopaedias, web pages, parallel texts, and field experts.
3) Genre	Parallel texts in the target language and genre, normative documents that define the genre, and field experts.
4) General language usage	Grammars, manuals of style, writing guides, and so forth.

Figure 6.2. Types of information needed
in the translation process and resources for each

Planning and organizing preparatory research

When we are faced with translating a highly specialized text on an unfamiliar topic, it is always advisable to spend time researching the subject matter before launching into the task of reading and making sense of the text. If the subject matter is already familiar, then before embarking on any checks or searches or consulting any documents, the text should be read very thoroughly. This is important for two reasons. Firstly, because we can then limit any searches to what is strictly necessary; spending a little longer on a careful reading of the text can often save a good deal of time. Secondly, it is only after a detailed reading that we can determine exactly what type of information we still need to acquire.

Once the specific needs analysis has been done, we are then ready to look for solutions, initially probably in documentary sources. If all else fails, we can, of course, consult experts in person, though this generally requires greater effort and is more time-consuming.

Document searches should be carried out in a sensible and coherent order, consulting initially well-known, easily accessible works. Printed sources – and their digitized on-line versions, which usually cost money – often provide more reliable information than free websites. Although printed works may contain less information, it is likely to be more detailed than that found on many free websites; these, on the other hand, do have the added advantage of being (sometimes!) regularly updated. Information available on websites, however, is often hastily assembled, roughly put together and sometimes poorly expressed and may have a somewhat "provisional" feel to it. So, we have plenty of resources available, but need to choose wisely from among them.

Printed sources and their digitized versions	Free www sources
• Less accessible • Authorship is normally more reliable • Less up-to-date • Less information but of better quality • More established knowledge • Less versatile format when doing searches and building minicorpora	• More accessible • Authorship is normally less reliable and often unknown • Normally more up-to-date • More information but often of worse quality • More provisional knowledge • More versatile format when doing searches and building minicorpora

Figure 6.3. Advantages and disadvantages of different types of information sources

Searching in data bases

Data bases such as *Medline* or *Excerpta Medica-EMBASE* are precious tools when translating highly specialized medical texts. When selecting a suitable data base, bear in mind the following aspects:

- *International coverage.* Some data bases are more international than others. For example, *Medline* has a broad international coverage of many topics.
- *Topic.* Some data bases cover just one specialized field, such as *Sports*, whereas others are multidisciplinary, as is the case of *Scirus*.
- *Languages.* Although the abstracts are normally published in English to promote international communication, national data bases give access to full articles written in their respective languages. National data bases are useful as sources of parallel texts to support the writing of the target text.
- *Genres.* Some data bases include just research genres such as original articles, scientific editorials, revision articles, and so forth, whereas others also include other genres published outside research journals. For example, *Dissertation Abstracts* includes theses.
- *Time.* Some data bases cover longer periods of time than others.

In data bases we can basically do two types of searches: precise searches, which allow us, for example, to analyze the phraseology and abbreviated forms of a given term; and exhaustive searches, which allow us, for example, to read about a topic we are interested in.

6.2 Starting up your own medical translation library

The following resources have been conceived of as a starting point from which to build your own medical translation library. (NB: the links in this section were last accessed some months before the publication of this book. Since the www is constantly changing, some of the less stable links may not be active by the time you try to access them.)

Your medical translation library needs constant updating because new resources are put on the web everyday and what you add will depend on the type of work you do.

We have focused on resources in English since nowadays most medical information – both specialized and popular – is published in this language. However, we have also included some in major languages such as Spanish, German and French. If you work with other languages, you can use the resources below to help you in your search for and organization of information.

Introductions to health topics

The links below are especially useful for acquiring background knowledge on different medical specialties. They are also good sources of texts for classroom and on-line activities.

Hardin Library for the Health Sciences
   <http://www.lib.uiowa.edu/hardin/md>
Medical Encyclopedia (MedlinePlus)
   <http://www.nlm.nih.gov/medlineplus/encyclopedia.html>
Interactive Health Tutorials (MedlinePlus)
   <http://www.nlm.nih.gov/medlineplus/tutorial.html>
MedicineNet.com
   <http://www.medicinenet.com/script/main/hp.asp>
The Merck Manual of Medical Information
   <http://www.merck.com/mmhe/index.html>
The Merck Manual of Diagnosis & Therapy
   <http://www.merck.com/mrkshared/mmanual/home.jsp>
The Merck Manual of Health & Aging
   <http://www.merck.com/pubs/mmanual_ha/contents.html>
Reference.com Web Directory
   <http://www.reference.com/Dir/Health/Medicine>
Atlas of Human Anatomy in Cross Section
   <http://www.vh.org/adult/provider/anatomy/HumanAnatomy/Cross
   SectionAtlas.html>
Anatline
   <http://anatline.nlm.nih.gov/Anatline>
Wikipedia
   <http://www.wikipedia.org>
Essentials of Human Anatomy and Physiology
   <http://occawlonline.pearsoned.com/bookbind/pubbooks/marieb-essentials/
   chapter1/deluxe.html>
Gray's Anatomy of the Human Body
   <http://www.bartleby.com/107>
Net Anatomy
   <http://www.netanatomy.com>
WebAnatomy
   <http://www.msjensen.gen.umn.edu/webanatomy>
The Virtual Body
   <http://www.ehc.com/vbody.asp>
Tour of the Basics
   <http://gslc.genetics.utah.edu/units/basics/tour>
Biology Hypertextbook
   <http://web.mit.edu/esgbio/www>
3D Medical Animations Library
   <http://www.healthscout.com/nav/animation/68/main.html>

Anatomy & Physiology Animations, Movies & Interactive Tutorial Links
  http://science.nhmccd.edu/biol/ap1int.htm

Task 1. Acquiring introductory information about the subject matter of the text

You have accepted an assignment to translate a review article about peptic ulcer from English into your mother tongue. The text below is the abstract of the review.

1) Go to <http://www.nlm.nih.gov/medlineplus> and read introductory information about peptic ulcer and laparotomy in the links 'Health Topics' and 'Medical Encyclopaedia'.
2) Explore other resources in the list above to learn about these two concepts

Surgical management of peptic ulcer disease today – indication, technique and outcome.

AIMS: The current surgical management of peptic ulcer disease and its outcome have been reviewed. RESULTS: Today, surgery for peptic ulcer disease is largely restricted to the treatment of complications. In peptic ulcer perforation, a conservative treatment trial can be given in selected cases. If laparotomy is necessary, simple closure is sufficient in the large majority of cases, and definitive ulcer surgery to reduce gastric acid secretion is no longer justified in these patients. Laparoscopic surgery for perforated peptic ulcer has failed to prove to be a significant advantage over open surgery. In bleeding peptic ulcers, definitive hemostasis can be achieved by endoscopic treatment in more than 90% of cases. In 1-2% of cases, immediate emergency surgery is necessary. Some ulcers have a high risk of re-bleeding, and early elective surgery might be advisable. Surgical bleeding control can be achieved by direct suture and extraluminal ligation of the gastroduodenal artery or by gastric resection. Benign gastric outlet obstruction can be controlled by endoscopic balloon dilatation in 70% of cases, but gastrojejunostomy or gastric resection are necessary in about 30% of cases. CONCLUSIONS: Elective surgery for peptic ulcer disease has been largely abandoned, and bleeding or obstructing ulcers can be managed safely by endoscopic treatment in most cases. However, surgeons will continue to encounter patients with peptic ulcer disease for emergency surgery. Currently, laparoscopic surgery has no proven advantage in peptic ulcer surgery.

(Source: http://www.ncbi.nlm.nih.gov/entrez/query.fcgi?db=pubmed&list_
uids=10796046&cmd=Retrieve&dopt=Citation&indexed=google)

Printed specialized dictionaries and encyclopaedias

Monolingual specialized dictionaries are required when trying to understand com-
plex medical concepts. Among the most useful and reliable ones in English are:
Stedman's Medical dictionary. 26th ed. Baltimore: Williams & Wilkins; 1995.
Merriam-Webster's Medical Dictionary. Springfield: Merriam-Webster; 1995.
Dorland's Illustrated Medical Dictionary. 29th ed. Philadelphia: W-B Saunders;
    2000.
Mosby's Medical Dictionary, 7th ed. St. Louis: Mosby Elsevier; 2006.

Bilingual and multilingual medical dictionaries are used when writing the target
text:

Elsevier's Encyclopaedic Dictionary of Medicine. New York: Elsevier; 1988-
    1990.

When translating medical literature, we often come across terms that belong to
other scientific and technical fields. Hence the need to refer to dictionaries such
as:

Academic Press Dictionary of Science and Technology. San Diego: Academic
    Press; 1992.
McGraw-Hill Dictionary of Scientific and Technical Terms. 5th ed. New York:
McGraw-Hill; 1996.

In the translation of some genres we may have to deal with all kinds of terms
related to Statistics, Chemistry, Pharmacy. The following works and links may
be useful in this respect:

*How to Report Statistics in Medicine: Annotated Guidelines for Authors,
    Editors, and Reviewers.* T Lang and M Secic. Philadelphia: American College
    of Physicians; 1997.
*Pharmacological and Chemical Synonyms: A Collection of Names, Drugs,
    Pesticides & Other Compounds Drawn from the Medical Literature of the
    World.* 10th ed. EEJ Marler. Amsterdam: Excerpta Medica; 1994.
The Merck Index: An Encyclopedia of Chemicals, Drugs, and Biologicals.
    S Budavari, editor. 12th ed. Whitehouse Station: Merck Company; 1996.
SI Units for Clinical Measurements. DS Young and EJ Huth. Philadelphia:
    American College of Physicians; 1998.

Statistics.com
　　<http://www.statistics.com/content/onlinebooks.html>
Online Statistics Textbook
　　<http://davidmlane.com/hyperstat/>
Statistics Every Writer Should Know
　　<http://www.robertniles.com/stats>

On-line medical dictionaries

On-line Medical Dictionary (OMD) is a searchable dictionary created by Graham Dark and contains terms relating to biochemistry, cell biology, chemistry, medicine, molecular biology, physics, plant biology, radiobiology, science and technology. It contains over 46,000 definitions. Entries are cross-referenced to each other and to related resources elsewhere on the net.
<http://cancerweb.ncl.ac.uk/omd/index.html>

Merriam-Webster's Collegiate Dictionary
　　<http://www.m-w.com/dictionary>
MedlinePlus Medical Dictionary
　　<http://www.nlm.nih.gov/medlineplus/mplusdictionary.html>
Surgical/Medical Word Glossary (MT Desk)
　　<http://www.mtdesk.com/frame.php?frame=glossary>
MedTerms Medical Dictionary (Medicine Net)
　　<http://www.medicinenet.com/script/main/hp.asp>
Dorland's Medical Dictionary
　　<http://www.mercksource.com/pp/us/cns/cns_hl_dorlands.zQzpgzEzzSzp
　　pdocszSzuszSzcommonzSzdorlandszSzdorlandzSzdmd-a-b-000zPzhtm>
Online Medical Dictionary
　　<http://www.stedmans.com/section.cfm/45>
Petit lexique de termes médicaux
　　<http://www.biam2.org/dico.html>
Multilingual Glossary of technical and popular terms in nine European languages
(European Comission)
　　<http://users.ugent.be/~rvdstich/eugloss/welcome.html>
EURODICAUTOM (European Comission)
　　<http://europa.eu.int/eurodicautom/Controller>
Multilingual glossary of statistics terms (European Comission)
　　<http://europa.eu.int/comm/eurostat/research/index.htm>
Internet Glossary of Statistical Terms
　　<http://www.animatedsoftware.com/statglos/statglos.htm>
Statistics Glossary

<http://www.stats.gla.ac.uk/steps/glossary>
Glossary of Biotechnology for Food and Agriculture
   <http://www.fao.org/biotech/index_glossary.asp?lang=en>
Glossary of Research-Related Terms
   <http://www.urmc.rochester.edu/rsrb/pdf/glossary.pdf>
Life Science Dictionary
   <http://biotech.icmb.utexas.edu/search/dict-search.html>

Access to collections of on-line medical dictionaries

Medical On-line Dictionaries and Glossaries
   <http://www.interfold.com/translator/medsites.htm>
Your dictionary
   <http://yourdictionary.com/diction5.html#medicine>
A Web of On-line Dictionaries
   <http://www.facstaff.bucknell.edu/rbeard/diction.html>
Online Medical and Science Dictionaries
   <http://www.sciencekomm.at/advice/dict.html>
X-lation Medical Glossaries
   <http://xlation.com/glossaries/getglos.php?topic=medical&lang=all>
Online Medical & Bioscience Dictionaries, Glossaries and Terminologies
   <http://www.sciencekomm.at/advice/dict.html>
Medical Dictionaries, Glossaries and Terminology Alphabetical Site Index
   <http://www.medtrng.com/meddict.htm>
Glossaries of Genome / Human Genetics Terms
   <http://www.kumc.edu/gec/glossary.html#conditions>

Task 2: Finding definitions and equivalent terms

1) Go back to task 1 and extract the terms for your glossary.
2) Find a definition for each of them using the resources in this section. Write the source of the definition in brackets.
3) Find a translation in your target language using the resources in this section. Write the source of the term in the target language in brackets.

Term in the source language	Definition	Term in the target language
Endoscopic balloon dilatation		
Endoscopic treatment		
extraluminal ligation		

Gastric acid		
Gastric resection		
Gastroduodenal artery		
Hemostasis		
Laparotomy		
Peptic ulcer		

Gateways, search engines and directories

OMNI. *Organizing Medical Networked Information*
    <http://omni.ac.uk>
HealthWeb
    <http://healthweb.org>
MedWeb
    <http://www.medweb.emory.edu/MedWeb>
Medical Matrix
    <http://www.medmatrix.org>
Medscape
    <http://www.medscape.com>
Medem
    <http://www.medem.com>
Biosites
    <http://www.library.ucsf.edu/biosites>
Cliniweb International
    <http://www.ohsu.edu/cliniweb>
Elsevier
    <http://www.elsevier.com/wps/find/homepage.cws_home>
Accessmedicine
    <http://www.accessmedicine.com>
Science Direct
    <http://www.sciencedirect.com>
Scirus
    <http://www.scirus.com/srsapp>
Clinical Laboratory Science Internet Resources
    <http://members.tripod.com/~LouCaru/index-5.html>
Hardin Meta Directory of Internet Health Sources
    <http://www.lib.uiowa.edu/hardin/md>
Health A to Z
    <http://www.healthatoz.com>
Health Finder

<http://www.healthfinder.gov>
Healthkinks.Net
   <http://www.healthlinks.com>
Martindale's Health Science Guide
   <http://www.martindalecenter.com>
MedExplorer
   <http://ourworld.compuserve.com/homepages/futuremed/medexplr.htm>
MedHunt: Health On the Net Foundation
   <http://www.hon.ch>
MedNets
   <http://www.mednets.com>
Primary Care Internet Guide
   <http://www.uib.no/isf/guide/guide.htm>
Reuters Health Information
   <http://www.reutershealth.com/en>
Virtual Hospital
   <http://www.vh.org>
Medivista and *Metanex* (Deutche Medizin Forum)
   <http://www.medivista.de>
   <http://www.metanex.de>
Medknowledge (Dr. F Koc)
   <http://www.medknowledge.de>
Fisterra
   <http://www.fisterra.com>
Merck Source
   <http://www.mercksource.com/pp/us/cns/cns_home.jsp>
Nursing Resources
   <http://www.rtstudents.com/rnstudents>
MedicalStudent.com
   <http://www.medicalstudent.com>

On-line abbreviations and units of measurement

AcronymFinder
   <http://www.acronymfinder.com>
Dictionary of Units
   <http://www.ex.ac.uk/cimt/dictunit/dictunit.htm>
How Many?
   <http://www.unc.edu/~rowlett/units>
World Wide Web Acronym and Abbreviation Server
   <http://www.ucc.ie/info/net/acronyms/index.html>

Medical and Pharmaceutical Abbreviations Dictionary
<http://www.pharma-lexicon.com/medicalabbreviations.php>

In printed form, you can consult the following works:

Dictionary of Medical Acronyms and Abbreviations, 2nd ed. S Jablonski: Philadelphia: Hanley and Belfus; 1993.
The Davis book of medical abbreviations: A deciphering guide, SL Mitchell-Hatton. Philadelphia: Davis, 1991.
Stedman's abbreviations, acronyms and symbols. Baltimore: Williams and Wilkins, 1992.

Eponyms

Whonamedit.com
<http://www.whonamedit.com/index.cfm>

Drugs information

As mentioned in Chapter 7, there are three main ways of naming drugs: International Non-Proprietary Names, trade names and national names. Given the difficulties posed by the translation of the names of drugs, it is important to become familiar with sources of pharmaceutical information.

Center for Drug Evaluation and Research (Food and Drug Administration)
<http://www.fda.gov/cder/drug/default.htm>
Drugs information (MedlinePlus)
<http://www.nlm.nih.gov/medlineplus/druginformation.html>
EMEA – European Medicines Agency
<http://www.emea.eu.int/>
Medicines (World Health Organization)
<http://www.who.int/medicines/en/>
Electronic Medicines Compendium (Medicines.org.uk)
<http://emc.medicines.org.uk/>
DrugBank (University of Alberta)
<http://redpoll.pharmacy.ualberta.ca/drugbank/>
Pharmaceutical Company Directory (medi-lexicon). Searchable database of worldwide pharmaceutical companies where information about their products is provided.
<http://www.pharma-lexicon.com/pharmaceuticalcompanies.php>
Prescribing Information (RXmed)

<http://www.rxmed.com/b.main/b2.pharmaceutical/b2.prescribe.html>
Drug Guide (Infomed)
    <http://www.infomed.org/100drugs>
Drug Information Online
    <http://www.drugs.com/>

Information about international nomenclatures

In international scientific and technical communication it is sometimes necessary to use standardized terms. The following are basic references relevant to the
practice of medical translation. Although most of them are published in printed
form, in some you can find the same information free on the Internet.

Anatomy

Federative Committee on Anatomical Terminology (FCAT): *Terminologia
Anatomica. International Anatomical Terminology.* New York: Thieme, 1998.

Diseases

World Health Organization: *International statistical classification of diseases and
related health problems, 10th revision* (ICD-10). Geneve: WHO, 1992-1994. On-line
information about the *International Classification of Diseases* at:
    <http://www.who.int/classifications/icd/en/>

Pharmacy

World Health Organization: *International nonproprietary names (INN) for pharmaceutical substances. Cumulative list N° 10.* Geneve: OMS-WHO, 2002. [In Latin,
English, French, Russian and Spanish]

World Health Organization: *Lists of Recommended and Proposed INNs*
    <http://www.who.int/druginformation/general/innlists.shtml>
WHO Terminology Information System - INN-DCI
    <http://policy.who.int/cgi-bin/om_isapi.dll?infobase=wt99pha&softpage=B
    rowse_Whoterm_INN>
World Health Organization: *The use of stems in the selection of International
Nonproprietary Names (INN) for pharmaceutical substances* (2004)
    <http://whqlibdoc.who.int/hq/2004/WHO_EDM_QSM_2004.5.pdf>
World Health Organization: *ATC/DDD Index 2006*

<http://www.whocc.no/atcddd/indexdatabase/>
mSupply Support: *Alphabetical Listing of ATC drugs & codes* (2000)
    <http://www.msupply.org.nz/files/atc_alphabetical.pdf>
International Union of Pharmacology (IUPHAR): *Receptor Database*
    <http://www.iuphar-db.org/GPCR/index.html>
International Union of Pharmacology (IUPHAR): *Ion Channel Compendium*
    <http://www.iuphar-db.org/iuphar-ic/index.html>

Microbiology

International Committee on Systematic Bacteriology: *International code of nomenclature of bacteria: bacteriological code.* Washington: American Society for Microbiology, 1992. [In Latin] The same nomenclature can be found free at:
    <http://www.bacterio.cict.fr>, <http://www.dsmz.de/microorganisms/main.php?contentleft_id=14>, <http://wdcm.nig.ac.jp>.

International Committee on Taxonomy of Viruses: *Virus taxonomy: classification and nomenclature of viruses. Seventh report of the International Committee on Taxonomy of Viruses.* San Diego: Academic, 2000. [In Latin and English]

Biochemistry and Molecular Biology

International Union of Biochemistry and Molecular Biology (IUBMB): *Biochemical nomenclature and related documents: a compendium.* London: Portland, 1992. The same nomenclature can be found free at:
    <http://www.chem.qmul.ac.uk/iupac/bibliog/white.html>

International Union of Biochemistry and Molecular Biology (IUBMB): *Enzime nomenclature: recommendations 1992.* San Diego: Academic, 1992. The same nomenclature can be found free at:
    <http://www.chem.qmw.ac.uk/iubmb/enzyme>

Botany

International Botanical Congress. *International code of botanical nomenclature (Tokio Code). Regnum Vegetabile, n° 131.* Königstein: Koeltz, 1994. The same nomenclature can be found free in English, French, German and Slovak at:
    <http://www.bgbm.org/iapt/nomenclature/code/default.html>

Zoology

International Commission on Zoological Nomenclature: *International code of zoological nomenclature* (4th edition). London: International Trust for Zoological Nomenclature, 1999. [in Latin].

Information on terminological standardization

International Organization for Standardization:
    <http://www.iso.org/iso/en/ISOOnline.frontpage>
International Information Centre for Terminology:
    < http://www.infoterm.info>
Termnet. The International Network for Terminology:
    <http://linux.termnet.org>
European Committee for Standardization:
    <http://www.cenorm.be/cenorm/aboutus/index.asp>
Réseau international de néologie et de terminologie:
    <http://www.rint.org>
Centrum für internationale Terminologie und angewandte Linguistik:
    <http://cital.fh-konstanz.de>
American National Standards Institute:
    <http://www.ansi.org>

Free on-line medical research journals and textbooks

Free on-line medical journals and books in English, French, German, Spanish, Portuguese, Catalan, Czech, Danish, Italian, Lithuanian, Norwegian, Russian, Slovakian, Swedish, and Turkish. These are good sources of parallel texts.

FreeMedicalJournals.com
    <http://www.freemedicaljournals.com>
FreeBooks4Doctors.com
    <http://www.freebooks4doctors.com>

Dissertations

Digital dissertations. Although this data base covers US Universities, it also contains dissertations from some European Universities.
    <http://www.umi.com/dissertations>
Index to theses contains British and Irish dissertations.
    <http://www.theses.com>
Docthèses is a database containing French dissertations published by the Ministère de l'Enseignement Supérieur and the Agence Bibliographique de l'Enseignement Supérieur.

<http://www.chadwyck.com/products/basic_product_search.asp>
TESEO is published by the Spanish Ministerio de Educación y Cultura and contains the dissertations passed in Spanish Universities.
<http://www.mcu.es/TESEO/index.html>
Disonline.de. This Deutsche Bibliothek site collects information on digital dissertation projects in Germany.
<http://www.dissonline.de>

Institutions dealing with terminology

European Association for Terminology
<http://www.eaft-aet.net>
Unión Latina
<http://www.unilat.org>
RITerm
<http://www.riterm.net>
Nordterm
<http://www.tsk.fi/nordterm>
Joint Inter-Agency Meeting on Computer-Assisted Translation and Terminology
<http://jiamcatt.unsystem.org/english/jiamcate.htm>

Etymological dictionaries

Medical Terminology (University of Hong Kong) offers glossaries of Greek and Latin prefixes, suffixes and roots as well as exercises in medical terminology.
<http://ec.hku.hk/mt>
A Short Course in Medical Terminology (Des Moines University) offers glossaries of Greek and Latin prefixes, suffixes and roots as well as exercises in medical terminology.
<http://www.dmu.edu/medterms/>
Introduction to medical terminology offers a complete glossary of Greek and Latin roots, prefixes and suffixes with examples in English.
<http://www.mtworld.com/tools_resources/medical_terminology.html>

Guides for authors of research journals

Uniform Requirements for Manuscripts Submitted to Biomedical Journals: Writing & Editing for Biomedical Publication (International Committee of Medical Journal Editors)
<http://www.icmje.org>
Collection of links to instructions for authors of medical research journals
<http://mulford.mco.edu/instr/>

Style manuals and guides on how to write

The references in this subsection are especially relevant when translating, re-writing or revising research articles in English for publication in international journals.

Writing and Publishing in Medicine. 3rd ed. HJ Huth. Baltimore: Williams & Wilkins, 1999.
Successful scientific writing. A step-by-step guide for the biological and medical sciences. 2nd ed. JR Matthews, JM Bowen and RW Matthews. Cambridge: Cambridge University Press, 2000.
How to write a paper. 3rd ed. GM Hall editor. London: British Medical Journal Books, 2003.
Science and Technical Writing. A Manual of Style. 2nd ed. P Rubens editor. New York: Routledge, 2001.
The Chicago Manual of Style. 14th ed. Chicago: University of Chicago Press, 1993.
Resources for Medical Writers (Medical Writing)
    <http://www.writerswrite.com/medical/medlink.htm>
Writing and Presenting Scientific Work (MedBioWorld)
    <http://www.sciencekomm.at/advice/presenting.html>

Patents

When dealing with assignments about genetic engineering, cloning, and drugs we may need to do searches in patent databases:
Delphion contains European, Japanese and American patents in different languages:
    <http://www.delphion.com>.

On-line data bases

Medline is the biggest medical data base and it can be extremely useful in medical translation practice. From *PubMed* (the interface created to use Medline): 1) you have free access to all abstracts in *Medline*; 2) the abstracts give you access to the full documents, which are sometimes free; 3) each abstract is linked to other abstracts on the same or related topics; 4) when you do the search you can limit it to a specific genre.
    <http://www.ncbi.nlm.nih.gov/PubMed>

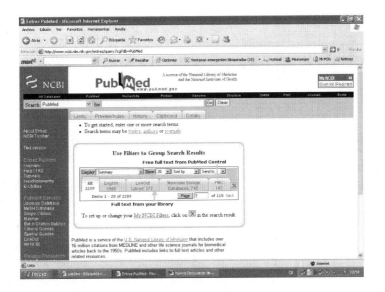

Figure 6.4. Pubmed, Medline's search engine

The Cochrane Library contains regularly updated evidence-based healthcare databases.

   <http://www.cochrane.org>

Medical Subject Heading (MeSH) consists of an alphabetical list and a tree structure. It is used by documentalists as a international classification tool for medical information. It can also be very useful for translators as a semantic and terminological tool.

   <http://www.nlm.nih.gov/mesh/meshhome.html>

A	Anatomy
B	Organisms
C	Diseases
D	Chemical & Drugs
E	Analytical, Diagnostic & Therapeutic Techniques & Equipment
F	Psychiatry & Psychology
G	Biological Sciences
H	Physical Sciences

I	Anthropology, Education, Sociology & Social Phenomena
J	Technology, Industry, Agriculture
K	Humanities
L	Information Science
M	Persons
N	Health Care
Z	Geographic locations

Figure 6.5. MeSH categories

C1	Bacterial Infections & Micoses
C2	Virus Diseases
C3	Parasitic Diseases
C4	Neoplasms
C5	Musculoskeletal Diseases
C6	Digestive Systems Diseases
C7	Stomatognathic Diseases
C8	Respiratory Tract Diseases
C9	Otorhinolaryngologic Diseases
C10	Nervous System Diseases
C11	Eye Diseases
C12	Urologic & Male Genital Diseases
C13	Female Genital Diseases & Pregnancy Complications
C14	Cardiovascular Diseases
C15	Hemic & Lymphatic Diseases
C16	Neonatal Diseases & Abnormalities
C17	Skin & Connective Tissue Diseases
C18	Nutritional & Metabolic Diseases

C19	Endocrine Diseases
C20	Immunologic Diseases
C21	Injuries. Poisoning & Occupational Diseases
C22	Animal Diseases
C23	Symptoms & General Pathology

Figure 6.6. Subcategories of diseases in MeSH

The Medical Subject Index (MeSH) is an index organized hierarchically by topic. Thus the broadest concept in the list below is the one at the top , "Digestive System Diseases", coded C06. As we go down the list, the terms refer to a more specific part of the digestive system and the code shows this. Thus the term "Peptic ulcer" (used in tasks 1 and 2 above) appears near the bottom of the list with the code C06.405.469.275.800.

Digestive System Diseases [C06]
Gastrointestinal Diseases [C06.405]
Intestinal Diseases [C06.405.469]
Duodenal Diseases [C06.405.469.275]
Duodenal Neoplasms [C06.405.469.275.270]
Duodenal Obstruction [C06.405.469.275.395] +
Duodenitis [C06.405.469.275.600]
Duodenogastric Reflux [C06.405.469.275.700]
Peptic Ulcer [C06.405.469.275.800]
Duodenal Ulcer [C06.405.469.275.800.348]
Peptic Ulcer Perforation [C06.405.469.275.800.698]

Figure 6.7. MeSH tree structures
Source: <http://www.nlm.nih.gov/cgi/mesh/2006/MB_cgi>

Embase is a comprehensive pharmacological and biomedical database renowned for extensive indexing of drug information from 4,550 journals published in 70 countries.
    <http://www.embase.com>

Current Contents Search provides users with the most up-to-date research information by means of unlimited access to tables of contents and bibliographic data from over 7,600 of the world's leading scientific and scholarly journals and 2,000 books.

Science Citation Index provides access to current and retrospective bibliographic information, author abstracts, and cited references found in 3,700 of the world's leading scholarly science and technical journals covering more than 100 disciplines.

Journal Citation Reports presents quantifiable statistical data that provides a systematic, objective way to evaluate the world's leading journals and their impact and influence in the global research community.

BIOSIS databases integrate citations for articles, meetings, patents, book chapters, and so on, about subjects from many different fields in biology.

Chemical Abstracts database includes over 20 million citations to the worldwide literature of chemistry and its applications from 1967 onwards. Producer: Chemical Abstracts Service, American Chemical Society.

PsycINFO The American Psychological Association's PsycINFO database is the comprehensive international bibliographic database for psychology. It contains citations and summaries of peer-reviewed journal articles, book chapters, books, dissertations, and technical reports, all in the field of psychology and the psychological aspects of related disciplines, such as medicine, psychiatry, nursing, sociology, education, pharmacology, physiology, linguistics, anthropology, business, and law. Journal coverage, spanning 1872 to present, includes international material selected from more than 1,900 periodicals written in over 35 languages.

ChemID is a database of chemical synonyms, structures, regulatory list information, and links to other databases containing information about the chemicals.
    <http://chem.sis.nlm.nih.gov/chemidplus>
HSRPROJ (Health Services Research Projects in Progress) is a database providing access to ongoing grants and contracts in health services research.
    <http://www.nlm.nih.gov/hsrproj>
TOXLINE Toxicology Literature Online.
    <http://toxnet.nlm.nih.gov/cgi-bin/sis/htmlgen?TOXLINE>
TOXNET Databases on toxicology, hazardous chemicals, environmental health, and toxic releases.
    <http://toxnet.nlm.nih.gov/cgi-bin/sis/htmlgen?index.html>

Organizations that distribute medical information

In this subsection your attention is drawn to all kinds of patients' associations; international, national and local official institutions devoted to health, such as scientific societies, ministries, hospitals, etc.; professional organizations of nurses, physicians, psychologists, etc.; University departments; pharmaceutical laboratories; publishing houses; research groups; and so on. One of the most important health organizations worldwide is the *World Health Organization (WHO)*:

    <http://www.who.int>.

German National Library of Medicine

    <http://www.zbmed.de>

Deutches Institut für Medizinische Dokumentation und Information (German Health Ministry)

    <http://www.dimdi.de>

Virtual library of the University of Düsseldorf

    <http://www.uni-duesseldorf.de/WWW/ulb/mezeit.html>

Medical associations

British Medical Association

    <http://www.bma.org.uk/ap.nsf/content/home>

American Medical Association

    <http://www.ama-assn.org>

The Bundesärztekammer (German Medical Association)

    <http://www.bundesaerztekammer.de>

Organización Médica Colegial de España (Spanish Medical Association)

    <http://www.cgcom.org>

Public institutions

World Health Organization

    <http://www.who.int>

European Union

    <http://europa.eu.int/pol/health/index_en.htm>

National Institutes of Health

    <http://www.nih.gov>

Food and Drug Administration

    <http://www.fda.gov>

6.3 Searching the web

The danger of information overload

It has never before been so easy to get hold of readily available information on every conceivable topic. The Internet offers any user endless free information which only a few years ago would not even have been available to the most privileged members of society. Besides this, we have at our disposal an ever-increasing number of wide-ranging scientific publications and research journals, many of which are available on-line. This vast store of readily-accessible knowledge has radically changed the way translators work and has made the job of technical and scientific translation much easier.

Nevertheless, this superabundance of information has its downside. We can easily be overwhelmed by the sheer volume of it and if we are not careful much of our precious time can be wasted sorting the wheat from the chaff.

In addition, greater care must be taken when using the Internet rather than published material because much of what circulates is not evaluated. For example, University of Pennsylvania researchers accessed the first 250 carpal tunnel syndrome web sites identified by five commonly used search engines. Among the 250 web sites, 75 were duplicated and 175 were unique. Fourteen percent (25) of the 175 web site addresses had misleading content; nine percent (16) presented unconventional information; and 31 percent (54) had non-informational content. So beware!

In view of this, we require a method which will enable us to find what we need effectively and efficiently. The criteria we should bear in mind are:

Needs

This really needs no further comment. It should be obvious by now that the more precisely our needs are defined, the sooner we shall be able to locate what is useful without being sidetracked by interesting curiosities or frustrated by entering blind alleys.

Reliability

The reliability of a document depends on whether the information it contains is truthful, strictly accurate and up-to-date and all this is largely a function of where it originates and who wrote it. Unfortunately, although the quantity of available information is vast, the quality often leaves much to be desired and translators should exercise caution in their use of websites. Linguistic quality can often be an indication of content quality.

Formal quality

Grammar, spelling, syntax, style, vocabulary, typography, and visual presentation are often indicative of the overall quality of a web page.

Accessibility

Libraries of printed works are rarely the first places translators go for information. Our first port of call is usually the Internet. However, the massive increase in websites accessible only to subscribers and the uncontrolled growth of websites in general have made many search engines obsolete or inefficient. Nowadays, even the best search engines are capable of locating less than half of the information available.

Time

For professional translators, time is of the essence and reducing as far as possible the hours spent both on translating and on searching for information is the number one priority. Success depends on the methods we use, the efficiency of search engines and the degree to which we are able to define our needs.

For ease of use, these criteria can be summarized in the following questions:

---

1. Have you done a needs analysis?
2. Does the text specifically relate to your question?
3. Is the webpage easily accessible?
4. Is the author clearly identified by name?
5. Are there any links to commercial companies that might involve bias?
6. Is the document associated with an institution which has some authority?
7. Is it clear when the document was created?
8. Is it up-to-date and is there evidence of its being frequently revised?
9. Is the data relatively recent?
10. Is the webpage well written and properly presented?

Figure 6.8. Criteria for evaluating web pages

Task 3. Evaluating web sites

Have a look at the following web sites. Evaluate them using questions 3-9 in Figure 6.8. One is good, the other one not so good (the url will give you a hint).

A. <http://www.montana.edu/craigs/Goal%20Orient%20art.htm>
B. <http://www.tucsonweekly.com/tw/01-14-99/cin.htm>

Types of search

Search by topic

These are carried out by consulting subject directories, such as those available at *Yahoo* <http://www.yahoo.com> or *Altavista* <http://www.altavista.com>. The catalogues are arranged from the most general to the most particular. For example, if we need information about methods of certification in organic farming, we go to the first page of Yahoo and select the category which might contain what we require: Science and Technology. This brings up a list of more specific categories and we continue thus until we find the documents we need. Remember that these search engines will not reveal all the information on a specific topic stored on the web and may not always be presented coherently.

Example of search by topic using Yahoo's directory

1. Home
2. Home > Science
3. Home > Science > Agriculture
4. Home > Science > Agriculture > Organic Farming
5. Home > Science > Agriculture > Organic Farming > Certification
6. Home > Science > Agriculture > Organic Farming > Certification > U.S. National Organic Program

---

Figure 6.9. Example of search by topic

Search by organization

Knowing the URL of the website of an organization related to the theme of our text allows us to go directly to the information. For translating medical texts, it may be useful to consult the website of the World Health Organization. All we need to do is type the address <http://www.who.org> in the browser. Collecting useful URLS and storing them properly can save time and effort in the future.

Search by key words

This is probably the most common. At the time of writing, *Google* is the most rapid and efficient search engine. In order to refine the results, search engines use Boolean operators: AND (conjunction), OR (disjunction) and NOT (negation). The combination of Boolean operators and literal text (sequences of words in quotation marks) gives the most useful search refinements. Nevertheless, each search engine has its own variations on advanced search which we need to know to get the best results.

6.4 Using parallel texts

Parallel texts are the texts we use in the consultation process in which we find solutions to a variety of problems.

Translators deal with real acts of communication, and hence encounter problems for which there are seldom established solutions. Beyond terminology, we have to deal with a variety of issues – such as tenor, modality, phraseology, preferences of the client, and so forth – for which there are no repertories of established equivalences, such as bilingual dictionaries. But even on matters of terminology, the solutions to particular problems in real assignments are not always to be found in dictionaries or glossaries, either because we are dealing with newly formed terms or because there are several synonyms for the same term and the choice depends on the specific target context, text and even client.

We can often find solutions to these kinds of problems in parallel texts. Parallel texts range from encyclopaedic articles to texts belonging to the genre of the target text, such as research article, report, scientific letter, patient's information leaflet, clinical protocol, patient's history, patent, and so on. Once we have found suitable parallel texts, we analyze them and finally extract solutions to solve problems.

We use parallel texts to understand the source text and or to write the target text. Imagine the following situation: we are reading a text on a topic that we are not familiar with. We look up the definitions of key terms in a specialized dictionary and yet we still don't understand them enough because we lack the conceptual background in that subject. Instead of trying to grasp the meaning of terms by means of definitions from a specialized dictionary, we may follow a different strategy: reading an introductory text about the same topic aimed at a more general audience. Since at this stage we are just interested in acquiring background conceptual knowledge, the language of the text will not really matter.

Parallel texts can also be used to help us to understand the sense of particular terms in particular contexts and therefore to select the appropriate meaning in any given situation.

From the point of view of the target text, parallel texts can be used to find terminological equivalents and to validate terminological equivalents previously found in dictionaries or glossaries. Neologisms may not yet be included in dictionaries but parallel texts originally written in closely related languages can be inspiring when we are trying to find the right word in the target language. When translating a new medical term into Spanish, the solutions found in parallel texts in Catalan, Italian, French or Portuguese might give us a clue if not a definitive solution.

Parallel texts are tools which help us to become aware of key aspects of target text production such as tenor, modality, phraseological patterns, prototypical macrostructure and extension of target genre, terminological and stylistic preferences of the client, and so on, and to discover the conventions expected by the readership of a particular genre in a specific context.

Parallel texts may be written originally in the source language, the target language or any other language, and they may or may not belong to the same genre as the target text. When translating a document for the approval of a drug in the target country, we will need to comply with the norms of the genre in he target jurisdiction and it will be necessary to analyze a text of that genre originally written in the target language in order to extract information relevant to sections of the document, legal requirements, and so on.

Sometimes we even need to comply with the explicit or implicit norms of a particular organization in order to write a fully acceptable translation. For example, if we are translating a press release for the World Health Organization, the best parallel text to solve target text production problems will be one not just of the same genre, but also published by the WHO.

Bear in mind the following aspects:

- *Subject matter:* the closer the subject matter of the parallel text to that of the source text, the better;
- *Quality of information and text:* date and author define the reliability of the information contained in the parallel text; the author may also be indicative of the quality of the language of the text; the degree of specialization of the information has to be in accordance with our needs;
- *Original language of parallel text:* when trying to solve linguistic problems relating to the target text, it is important to use texts originally written in the target language.
- *Target genre:* in order to solve target text production problems – such as prototypical length and macrostructure – , the parallel text should belong to the target genre;
- *Preferences of client:* this is a key strategic aspect governing the acceptability of the target text.

A word of caution

Of course not all parallel texts on the Internet are of acceptable quality. Those who write on health matters are seldom professional writers, and many of them don't write in a language they master fully. Besides, many are translations in a more or less direct way, and they may contain the defects of non-professional translation. Translators must take these factors into account and use parallel texts with caution. The fact that a parallel text contains a possible solution does not mean that it is the best solution or even that it is a solution at all. Three strategies can be followed when the quality of the parallel text is not clear enough: validate the solutions in other parallel texts; use *Google* to see the frequencies of use of a particular solution (bearing in mind that people can be wrong!); and consult a subject expert.

Task 4. Using parallel texts

In chapter 2, ten medical genres are explored from a communicative and formal point of view.

1) Choose one of them and find three examples of it originally written in your target language that deal with the same or similar topic. To find them, you can use the references provided in chapter 2. You can also use Google – or any other search engine – advanced options.
2) Find a text in English belonging to the genre you have chosen and dealing with the same topic. Your assignment will be to translate it into your target language.
3) As you translate it, read the three parallel texts for possible solutions to the problems you come across.
4) Explain which parallelisms you can find between the parallel texts originally written in your target language and your target text.

6.5 Collaboration of subject matter experts and other translators

When we cannot find what we need in documents, we turn to subject matter experts and other, more experienced, translators. This is especially true for translators without a solid medical background. But even health professionals who earn their living as translators frequently consult others since nowadays no health professional can cover in depth all existing medical specialities.

As we mentioned in chapter 1, medical translation is an interdisciplinary professional practice. It involves management of medical knowledge and participation in communication processes within and between communities of the various health sectors (patients, physicians, nurses, researchers, general public, University lecturers and students, etc.) in specific contexts: hospitals, laboratories, official institutions, etc. Knowing the way communication takes place in these communities and contexts is extremely important. Through the collaboration of subject matter experts, the medical translators not only have access to particular solutions for particular assignments, but they are also able to socialize with the members of the knowledge community in which their translations will eventually be used.

Subject matter experts can be approached either directly through personal contact, or indirectly using on-line resources such as virtual communities, distribution lists, and sites of professional associations, University departments, patients' associations, research teams, and so on. At <http://bio.hgy.es> the *Red Universitaria de Servicios Telemáticos Integrados para Comunidades Virtuales de Usuarios* (UNINet) provides an international collection of virtual communities in the biomedical fields.

There are some very active international virtual communities of medical translators on the Internet:

Medical Translators
   <http://health.groups.yahoo.com/group/medical_translation>
Medtrad. Besides having a very active distribution list, *Medtrad* also publishes a journal on the practice of medical translation called *Panace@*.
   <http://www.medtrad.org>

For a list of groups dealing with health matters such as nutrition, reproductive medicine, alternative medicine, or drugs and medications, consult *Yahoo*'s directory *Health & Wellness* at <http://health.dir.groups.yahoo.com/dir/Health_ Wellness>.

The collaboration of subject matter experts or other translators can be useful on different fronts: getting to understand complex concepts of the source text; finding reliable sources of information of all kinds, from images to dictionaries; finding solutions for terms and expressions that don't appear in dictionaries; acquiring a very accurate idea of how the target text will be used, for what purposes, by whom, and in what situations. Subject matter experts are particularly useful as ideal readers of our translations and their comments on the finished target text are very valuable.

When communicating with subject matter experts it is important to remember that you belong to different professional communities and have different backgrounds. The subject matter expert is not familiar with the terminology of translation: source text, target text, genre, equivalence, function, technique, modulation, and so on. Thus avoid jargon and be as clear as possible. It is also important that before asking for personal help, you do some background work on the problems you want to solve so that the questions you ask are focused. When the communication takes place on-line, it is particularly important to avoid mis-understandings of all kinds. And always remember to thank your helper.

A word of caution

Different subject matter experts or experienced translators may have diverging views on the same problem or solution. What subject experts regard as acceptable may be perfectly so in their own working context, but not in the working context of the target text you are writing. The safest approach is to check solutions with other experts or by means of *Google*.

Subject experts − especially researchers − are used to reading biomedical literature in English. This exposure to English means that they often have syntactic and lexical interferences in their mother tongues which translators should be aware of.

Subject matter experts may have pre-conceived ideas about what a good translatioin is. These ideas may or may not coincide with the functionalist approach that underlies most professional translation practice.

Finally, not all subject experts have the same degree of competence and experience in their specialities and therefore the reliance we can place on their opinions may vary.

Task 5. Working with a subject matter expert

The purpose of this task is that you socialize with a subject matter expert so that you can receive her/his help in the translation process, can understand the possible information requirements of that particular professional, and can grasp some of the norms of the knowledge community to which s/he belongs. Translate a text that can be useful for the subject matter expert in her/his professional environment so that both of you benefit from the task.

1) Find someone who is professionally involved in the health sector: a physician, a nurse, a surgeon, a dentist, a physiotherapist, a psychologist, a psychiatrist, a biomedical researcher, a pharmacist, or any other health professional.
2) Find out what type of knowledge they use in their professional practice.

> 3) Find a text that is of her/his professional interest.
> 4) Translate it into your target language.
> 5) Ask for help from the subject matter expert in aspects such as understanding difficult concepts, using information sources, using terminology in the target language, and revising the final version.

6.6 Further tasks

Task 6. Using different search engines

1) Using *Yahoo*'s, *Altavista*'s and *Google*'s directories, find resources of medical information in your mother tongue.
2) Compare the results from the three directories.

Task 7. Exploring parallel texts

1) Choose a specialized text on any medical field in your mother tongue.
2) Find a text in English of the same characteristics: topic, genre, date, etc.
3) Read them carefully and extract the conceptual and formal paralellisms that you find in them.

Task 8. Using Medline

1) Choose a research article from any journal at <http://www.fremedicaljournals.com>.
2) Using *Medline*'s *PubMed*, find the following information about the key terms of the article: definitions (or part of the definitions), word combinations in which they appear (collocational patterns), synonyms and abbreviated forms, if any.

6.7 Further reading

Austermühl, Frank (2001) *Electronic Tools for Translators*, Manchester: St. Jerome.

Lee-Janhke Hannelore (2001) 'L'enseignement de la traduction médicale: un double défi?', *Meta* 46(1): 145-153.

Morton L. and S. Godbolt (1992) (eds) *Information Sources in the Medical Sciences*, London: Bowker-Saur.

Roper F.W. and J.A. Borkman (1994) (eds) *Introduction to reference sources in the health sciences*, Metuchen (NJ): Medical Library Association.

Tilley C. (1990) 'Medical databases and health information systems', *Annual Review of Information Science and Technology* 25: 313-382.

Winker, M.A. (2000) 'Guidelines for Medical and Health Information Sites on the Internet', *Journal of the American Medical Association* 238(12). Available at: <http://jama.ama-assn.org/issue/v283n12/full/jsc00054.html>.

7. Dealing with terms and other units of specialized knowledge

> The Greek forms provided the model for scientific terminology in Europe; they were translated into Latin (which was fairly close to Greek both in its grammatical structure and its semantic organisation), and the Latin terms were subsequently borrowed into the modern European languages.
>
> M.A.K. Halliday (1998: 199)

Overview of chapter

We create medical terms by means of linguistic procedures in specific historical and cultural conditions (7.1). From Greek and Latin we have inherited the basic combining forms that constitute the core of scientific medical terminology in any language (7.2). Two general tendencies of relevance for the translator can be observed in terminological development: one towards standardization and unification (7.3), the other towards variation and innovation (7.4). They are the two sides of the same coin: the two are complementary and the translator should ignore neither. Sometimes we may be required to avoid technical terminology in the writing of the target text so that non-specialists can understand its content (7.5). Some tasks (7.6) and suggestions for further reading (7.7) are given at the end of the chapter.

7.1 Terminologizing medical knowledge

By terminologizing we understand establishing concepts and naming them. As new diseases appear and biomedical research advances, new knowledge is generated, which has to be conceptualized and transmitted. Thus, the purpose of terminologizing medical knowledge is to organize it, store it and make it available for communication. Think of eponymy, one of the most visible ways of naming anatomical parts, botanical genera, diseases, syndromes, theories, tests, or procedures: Vesalius ligament, Graafian follicle (discovered by De Graaf), Parkinson's disease, Bechterew's arthritis, Bernard-Horner syndrome, Wernicke-Korsakoff syndrome, Castaneda's method, Watson-Crick helix, etc.

Things out there or inside us have not always had a name. In fact, many of them still don't have names either because we don't know they exist yet or because so far the need to refer to them has not arisen. As we discover or invent them, we attach names to them. And we do it by means of the resources of our language. One of the most challenging aspects of the activity of medical writers and translators has always been to find (and agree on) ways of naming new phenomena.

The process of terminologizing medical knowledge as the need arose began at least twenty-five centuries ago. As we will see in the next section, we have inherited a vast number of Greek and Latin terms created to respond to the ever-growing store of knowledge about health and disease. Since the time of Hippocrates, discoveries and inventions in any medical field have required specific words to name them. Here is a recent example.

In the 1970s nobody knew about AIDS. In fact, the acronym AIDS did not exist. Yet many people are thought to have died of AIDS related illnesses during that decade. The first recognized cases of AIDS occurred in the USA in the early 1980s. The data for the first reports of an 'unusual epidemic' with excess morbidity in certain gay communities of the US were examined by researchers at the Danish Cancer Institute in collaboration with researchers from Bethesda, Maryland as early as 1979. At this time AIDS did not yet have a name. It was a completely unknown epidemic. The discovery of the Human Immunodeficiency Virus made clear that it was the cause of the syndrome, which, as a consequence, was named Acquired Immune Deficiency Syndrome (AIDS).

The mechanisms of terminologization

One of the most common and productive ways in which new terms are created is referred to by linguists as nominalization. In this process, verb phrases (or less frequently adjectival phrases) are transformed into noun phrases. Compare the following sentences (quoted from Halliday, 1998: 191):

1. The driver drove the bus too rapidly down the hill, so the brakes failed
2. The driver's overrapid downhill driving of the bus resulted in brake failure

Notice that the differences between the two sentences are not in meaning, nor in lexical items, but in grammatical categories. The sequence "the brakes failed" in (1) becomes "brake failure" in (2). This category shift is called "grammatical metaphor". Such transformations are the basis of the development of scientific terminologies.

What we do through grammar is to transform our experience into meaning. The grammar allows us to create a universe of objects and relations, imposing categories on our perceptions of phenomena. Rather than simply reflecting or codifying something that is already given in nature, the grammar imposes categorizations, that is, particular ways in which the phenomena of our experience can be seen to be related one another.

The power of transforming categories is inherent in grammar and allows us to distil scientific meaning and create taxonomies of objects and processes. Take a look at the following example:

bodies move > the body is moving > a moving body > the body's moving > the movement of bodies > body motion > kinesis > bradykinesia, etc.

This process of distillation culminates in the medical terms bradykinesia, akinesia, dyskinesia, etc. and is an example of the principle on which all medical terminology is ultimately based. Therefore, medical terminology is not an autonomous system separated from grammar, but exists thanks mainly to the nominalizing power of grammar.

Term = concept + denomination

As we have seen what the nominalizing power of grammar does is to distil meaning and establish conceptual categories. Thus, a term is formed by a concept – a distilled meaning that has been categorized – and a denomination – the external linguistic form.

Medical translators are interested in both components of the term. From the point of view of comprehension, we are especially interested in the concept represented by the denomination and the relationships between the main concepts on which the continuity of sense of the text is ultimately based, whereas for the production of the target text, we are more interested in the form or denomination of the term in the target language.

7.2 Greek and Latin basis of medical terms

In the last twenty-five centuries, modern languages have borrowed scientific terminology from Greek and Latin, mainly through the activity of translators. From this point of view, Greek and Latin are not dead languages. Some parts of them at least are still alive. This is especially true in medical terminology, as we shall see in this section.

In medicine the smallest unit relevant to meaning is not the word but the morpheme. More than five hundred roots, prefixes and suffixes form the basis of fundamental medical terminology. Their multiple combinations expand these initial forms to thousands of terms in most modern languages. And the use of Greek and Latin etymological forms still is and will continue to be one of the principal ways in which we can create, store and communicate new knowledge.

Many medical terms, old and new, are based on the same etymological forms (see Appendix 2). A knowledge of the Greek and Latin roots, prefixes and suffixes provides the basic building blocks of medical terminology and enables us to infer the meaning of the whole.

Task 1. Exploring etymological roots

The following terms indicate different types of inflammation. Find out what they mean using the etymological information of their roots. Use the information in Appendix 2 and the etymological information sources provided in Chapter 6.

Terms: arthritis, arteritis, bronchitis, carditis, cystitis, dermatitis, enteritis, gastroenteritis, glossitis, keratitis, laryngitis, lymphadenitis, mammitis, mastitis, myelitis, nephritis.

Task 2. Exploring etymological roots

The following terms indicate different types of treatment. Find out what they mean using the etymological information about their roots. Use the information in Appendix 2 and the etymological information sources provided in Chapter 6.

Terms: antibiotherapy, chemotherapy, hydrotherapy, immunotherapy, pneumotherapy, radiotherapy, thalassotherapy, thermotherapy.

Task 3. Exploring etymological prefixes and suffixes

The following terms contain the same root: hepat- (liver). Find their meaning using the etymological information of their suffixes. Use the information in Appendix 2 and the etymological information sources provided in Chapter 6.

Terms: hepatitis, hepatectomy, hepatoma, hepatoscopy, hepatoblastoma, hepatocarcinoma, hepatomegaly, hepatorrhagia, hepatotomy, hepatotoxin.

7.3 *In vitro* terminology: standardization

Think of the communicative activity carried out by international organizations such as the World Health Organization or by the pharmaceutical industry. Thousands of similar organizations both in the public and private sectors worldwide constantly need to standardize the terms they use, both within their own institutions and in order to bring themselves into line with other organizations so that international communication is made possible.

The globalizing tendency of the economy and communication together with the ever-growing number of medical terms require internationalized practices as far as terminology management is concerned. Two types of standardization practices can be distinguished: standardization of terminologies, and standardization of terminological principles and methods. International norms such as ISO/TC

37 'Terminology and language content resources' standardize basic principles, requirements and methods concerning terminology and language resources.

This section deals with classifications and nomenclatures, with other units of specialized knowledge (USKs) such as symbols and abbreviations representing concepts that are relevant to medical translation practice, and with translations of neologisms normalized by official organizations. They all reflect the tendency of terminology towards standardization.

Classifications and nomenclatures

With regard to terminology, scientific disciplines are well-organized corpora of concepts based on hierarchical classifications. Concepts and objects are ordered according to general criteria, and are grouped in categories or classes with common characteristics.

At this point it would be worth spending a few minutes exploring two of the world's largest systematized nomenclatures: the International Classification of Dieseases (ICD) (at http://www.who.int/classifications/icd/en), a World Health Organization classification which has become the international standard diagnostic classification for all general epidemiological and many health management purposes; and the Systematized Nomenclature of Medicine, which is rapidly gaining ground as the medical ontology worldwide. Its core terminology contains over 364,000 health concepts with unique meanings and formal logic-based definitions organized into hierarchies. It is available in English, Spanish, and German. It can be accessed at <http:www.snomed.org>.

Now let's consider at a couple of specific examples. The first one has been taken from the International Headache Society's International Classification of Headache:

> [...]
> 1. Migraine
> 2. Tension-type headache (TTH)
> 3. Cluster headache and other trigeminal autonomic cephalalgias
> 4. Other primary headaches
> 5. Headache attributed to head and/or neck trauma
>   [...]

The second one is from the Neuroepithelial Tumours of new WHO Classification of Tumours affecting the Central Nervous System:

[...]
7. Neuronal and mixed neuronal-glial tumors
   Gangliocytoma
   Dysplastic gangliocytoma of cerebellum (Lhermitte-Duclos)
   Ganglioglioma
   Anaplastic (malignant) ganglioglioma
   Desmoplastic infantile ganglioglioma
   desmoplastic infantile astrocytoma
   Central neurocytoma
   Dysembryoplastic neuroepithelial tumor
   Olfactory neuroblastoma (esthesioneuroblastoma)
   variant: olfactory neuroepithelioma
8. Pineal Parenchyma Tumors
   Pineocytoma
   Pineoblastoma
   Mixed pineocytoma/pineoblastoma
   [...]

For a discipline to be coherent each concept should be properly inserted in a classification and should have a name that represents it. The better established a discipline is, the more standardized is its terminology. Chemistry, Botany and Zoology are examples of scientific disciplines which have a long tradition of taxonomies and nomenclatures.

Nomenclatures are lists of terms that have been standardized and agreed on by a scientific community of experts of a particular discipline according to norms that determine their relationship with meaning. They form the conceptual core of any discipline or speciality. Thus they are not mere lists of terms arranged in alphabetical order. Rather nomenclatures are based on taxonomies and their basic organization is of a semantic nature.

Nomenclatures avoid synonymy, homonymy, polysemy, ambiguity and eponymy. Some of them are written in Latin, as is the case of Botany and Zoology. The purpose of nomenclature is twofold: the clarity and precision of communication, and the ease of information retrieval in information systems.

For the medical translator it is important to be aware of terminological standardization as a requirement of real assignments. The following nomenclatures are especially relevant to the medical translator since they correspond to disciplines closely related to biomedical research and practice or to biomedical specialities themselves: Chemistry, Botany, Bacteriology, Zoology, Anatomy, Virology, Genetics, Physiology, Immunology, International Non-proprietary names and Names of diseases.

Since nomenclatures and classifications are standardized terminologies developed by international organizations, translations into other languages are carefully controlled:

> Permission for translations must be applied for, and will be granted to National Headache Societies or Linguistic Groups of the International Headache Society. In the absence of a National Headache Society or Linguistic Group, a headache expert may be approved on behalf of the International Headache Society by the Chairman of the Headache Classification Subcommittee to be responsible for translation into a specific language. Sponsorships may be listed and advertisements accepted in translations. (<http://216.25.100.131/ihscommon/guidelines/pdfs/full_form_watermarked.pdf>)

A nomenclature of special importance for the medical translator is the International Nonproprietary Names for Pharmaceutical Substances (INN) published by the World Health Organization. However, this nomenclature has to compete with commercial names and national names for the same substance.

The WHO publishes the official international names of drugs in several languages: Latin, English, French, Spanish, and Russian. Take the following example:

Latin, English, French, Spanish	
Recommended INN *DCI Recommandée* *DCI Recomendada*	*Chemical name or description; Molecular formula; Graphic formula* *Nom chimique ou description; Formule brute; Formule développée* *Nombre químico o descripción; Fórmula empírica; Fórmula desarrollada*
adecatumumabum adecatumumab	immunoglobulin G1, anti-(human antigen 17-1A) (human monoclonal MT201 γ1-chain), disulfide with human monoclonal MT201 κ-chain, dimer

| adécatumumab | immunoglobuline G1, anti-(antigène 17-1A de la molécule d'adhésion de la cellule épithéliale humain) ; dimère du disulfure entre la chaîne γ1 et la chaîne κ de l'anticorps monoclonal humain MT201 |
| adecatumumab | inmunoglobulina G1, anti-(antígeno humano 17-1A) dímero del disulfuro entre la cadena γ1 y la cadena κ del anticuerpo monoclonal humano MT201 |

Figure 7.1. (WHO Drug Information, Vol. 18, No. 3, 2004)

Other units of specialized knowledge

Among other units of specialized knowledge of special interest for the translator are: abbreviations of medical terms, abbreviations of nucleic acids, abbreviations of chemical compounds, abbreviations of research journals, international system symbols, mathematical symbols, statistics symbols, vitamin symbols, chromosome symbols, gene symbols, symbols of malign tumours, etc. Translators should be familiar with all of them since they occur in the source text and will have to be dealt with in the target text.

Task 4. Dealing with abbreviations

Look at the following example taken from an abstract of a research article:

RESULTS: Significantly increased risks were found for deaths from tuberculosis (odds ratio (OR) 1.61, 95% confidence interval (CI) 1.23 to 2.11), chronic obstructive pulmonary disease (COPD) (OR 2.5, 95% CI 1.9 to 3.4), lung cancer (OR 4.8, 95% CI 2.9 to 8.0), other upper aerodigestive cancer (OR 3.0, 95% CI 1.9 to 4.9) and ischaemic heart disease (OR 1.7, 95% CI 1.2 to 2.3).

- Which expressions have been abbreviated? Why have they been abbreviated?
- How would you deal with them in your target language?

Some examples of common medical abbreviations and acronyms normally left in English when translating:

Abbreviation	Full form
ALCAPA	Anomalous left coronary artery from pulmonary artery
APNB	Alternating positive-negative pressure breathing
APUD	Amine and precursor uptake and decarboxilation
ASK	Antistreptokinase
AV	Atrioventricular
BAO	Basal acid output
BMR	Basal metabolic rate
BUN	Blood urea nitrogen
CFU	Colony-forming unit
CIG	Cold insoluble globulin
CMI	Cell-mediated-immunity
cRABP	Cytoplasmatic retinoic acid-binding protein
EAHF	Eczema, asthma, hay fever
ECT	Emission computed tomography
EGF	Epidermal growth factor
EPT	Electric response audiometry
FNAB	Fine needle aspiration biopsy
GH	Growth hormone
GRH	Growth releasing hormone
HDL	High density lipoprotein
HIV	Human immunodeficiency virus
ICSH	Interstitial cell-stimulating hormone
IFT	Immunofluorescence test
IM	Intramuscular
IV	Intravenous
LATS	Long-acting thyroid stimulator
LDL	Low density lipoproteins

LVF	Left visual field
MHC	Major histocompatibility complex
MCBF	Mast cell burst factor
NK	Natural killer
PAG	Pregnancy associated glycoprotein
PCR	Polymerase chain reaction
PSA	Prostate specific antigen
REM	Rapid eye movement
RVF	Right visual field
SMA	Smooth muscle antibodies
SPF	Specific pathogen free
TNF	Tumoral necrosis factor

Figure 7.2. Examples of common medical abbreviations

Some examples of common medical abbreviations normally left in Latin when translating:

Abbreviation	Latin phrase	Meaning
b.d.	Bis die	Twice a day
q.4.h.	Quaque 4 hora	Every four hours
alt.die	Alternus die	Every other day
alt.h.	Alternus horis	Every other hour
q.a.m.	Quaque ante meridiem	Every morning
q.n.	Quaque nocte	Every night
h.s.	Hora somni	At bed time
p.o.	Per os	Orally
s.l.	Sub linguam	Under the tongue
p.r.	Per rectum	Rectally
p.v.	Per vaginam	Vaginally
s.q.	Sufficiens quantitas	In sufficient quantity

Figure 7.3. Examples of common Latin abbreviations

Translations of neologisms normalized by official organizations

Standardization also takes place within particular languages. It normally occurs as a result of official linguistic policies aimed at promoting the use of that particular language, especially in scientific and technical fields. Authorities anxious to reinforce minority languages and cultures are particularly fond of this type of strategy. For example, the establishment and use of normalized translation of neologisms into French in Quebec is promoted officially by the *Office québécois de la langue française* <http://www.olf.gouv.qc.ca>. The same can be said of the Catalan government which encourages normalized translations of neologisms through a terminological office called *Termcat* <http://www.termcat.net>. The official academies of some languages are also responsible for overseeing normalized translations of neologisms in scientific and technical fields.

The translator's position vis a vis terminological standardization

Translators deal with real texts as acts of communication, not with nomenclatures as abstract systems. It is not their job to make people use nomenclatures in order to promote standardization but they will use nomenclatures if asked to do so in a given assignment.

One of the problems with nomenclatures is that they often produce terms that are not consistent with their own principles and criteria, or terms that are too long, difficult to pronounce, and difficult to memorize. However, the most important difficulties arise from the fact that standardized nomenclatures have to compete with popular and with traditional scientific terms. In fact, standardization is often not viable in translation practice.

A special case where the problems of applying nomenclatures are clearly seen is in the field of pharmaceutics. Although the WHO publishes a list of international non-proprietary names of drugs, often we find that source-text authors use either commercial or national common names.

As far as abbreviations are concerned, three recommendations may help: use approved forms in the target language; define – and explain if necessary – shortened forms at first mention; and pluralize correctly in the target language.

7.4 *In vivo* terminology: variation

Medical terminology is neither static nor uniform (one to one relationships between concept and linguistic form). Neither it is symmetric between languages. Even in anatomical terms, we find basic differences such as the way fingers and toes are named in English and in Spanish – 'dedos' for both – that affect the task of the translator.

Medical terminology changes in space (across languages and cultures) and time. As an example of the first type of variations, consider the following asymmetry: the English term 'anthrax' ('carbunco' in Spanish) does not correspond to the Spanish 'ántrax' ('carbuncle' in English). Besides, as pointed out by Navarro (2005: 192) the same concept can be found in texts in English referred to by a variety of words: charbon, splenic fever, malignant ulcer, woolsorter's disease, Siberian ulcer, malignant edema, ragsorter's disease and even the German calque milzbrand.

The second type of variations can be seen in terms such as 'neurosis' (originally denoting any disorder of the nervous system), melancholy (originally denoting black bile, *mélaina cholé* in Greek), or 'hysteria'(originally denoting a disease of the uterus, *hystéra* in Greek).

Even within the same language at any given time there is not always a fixed, one-to-one, straightforward relationship between words and the concepts they designate. Think of such a common term as 'drug', which can mean 'drug abuse', 'drug substance' and 'drug product' depending on the context.

In this section, we shall focus on important terminological features that have to do with intra and interlinguistic variation and change: morphology and spelling; language and culture; text and communicative situation; synonymy; polysemy; homonymy; false friends; neology; and updating of nomenclatures.

Morphology and spelling

Care should be taken with irregular plurals from Latin such as fungi, bacteria, cervix, thorax, ganglia, or data. When translating medical terms, special attention should be paid to the morphological variations in the endings of adjectives. Consider the following examples in three languages:

English	French	Spanish
Embryonal	Embryonnaire	Embrionario
Germinal	Germinative	Germinativo
Carpal	Carpien	Carpiano
Aortal	Aortique	Aórtico
Migrant	Migrateur	Migrador
Depressant	Dépressif	Depresivo
Coronary	Coronarien	Coronario
Flagellate	Flagellé	Flagelado
Calmative	Calmant	Calmante
Ulcerative	Ulcéreux	Ulcerativo, ulceroso
Appendiceal	Appendiculaire	Apendicular

Embolism	Embolie	Embolia
Olfactory	Olfactif	Olfatorio

Spelling variations from language to language of the same Greek and Latin roots, prefixes and suffixes should also be taken into account when translating, especially in sounds such as [f], [k], [s], and [i]: encephalitis, bradykinesia, cystectomy, haemorrhage, etc.

Language and culture

Different languages and cultures vary in the structure of medical terminology. One of the most obvious examples is the fact that some languages, such as English, have a double-layered medical vocabulary – that is, most scientific words have popular counterparts – whereas others, like Spanish or French, do not have them at all or do not have them to the same extent:

English	*French*	*Spanish*
Coagulation, clotting	Coagulation	Coagulación
Myopia, short-sightedness	Myopie	Miopía
Cicatrization, scarring	Cicatrization	Cicatrización

Inversely, Danish and Dutch have doublets where English hasn't:

Danish	*English*
Blindtarmsbetændelse, appendicitis	Appendicitis
Blindedarmontsteking, appendicitis	Appendicitis

This register mismatch (Pilegaard, 1997: 171) is one of the many terminological problems medical translators have to deal with. In this sense, the translator should be aware that what in Latin languages might sound too low a register is perfectly acceptable as scientific terminology in English:

English	*French*	*Spanish*
Birth defect	Malformation congénitale	Malformación congénita
One-egg twins	Jumeaux univitellins	Gemelos univitelinos
Growth of germs	Prolifération microbienne	Proliferación microbiana
Sweat canal	Canal sudorifère	Canal sudoríparo
Caked breast	Engorgement mammaire	Obstrucción mamaria
Taste buds	Papilles gustatives	Papilas gustativas

Medical terms in different languages and cultures do not always coincide. For example, terms such as schizophrenia, chronic bronchitis and peptic ulcer have different meanings in German, French and English (Pilegaard, 1997: 163). Likewise, the English amygdala does not coincide semantically with the Spanish 'amígdala'. Sometimes there is even lack of physical correspondence in different languages: French and German have no terms for knuckle, and Russian has no distinction between hand and arm.

Text and communicative situation

The characteristics of the particular text to be translated and the communicative situation in which it is embedded determine not only the style and the pragmatic elements, but also the choice of terms in the target language. Thus terminological choice when there is more than one word to name the same concept often varies according to the conventions of the genre to which the target text belongs. The same concept may be represented by different words in a research article, in a patient's history, in a newspaper article and in a patient's information brochure. This aspect is especially relevant when translating across genres, that is, when the target genre is not the same as the source genre due to the demands of the particular assignment.

Public and private organizations in the health sector have different preferences and habits as far as terminology is concerned. For example, the terminological preferences and habits of the World Health Organization as far as naming drugs is concerned are different from those of drug companies. Discovering these preferences by means of parallel texts is a key strategy we make use of in order to write translations whose terminology is perfectly acceptable to the client and the final reader of the text.

Synonymy

One of the commonest forms of variation in medical terminology is the existence of more than one word to express the same concept. Synonyms are frequent in medical texts. They may be a cause of confusion for the translator both in the comprehension of the source text and the writing of the target text. Hence, the importance of becoming aware of the main sources of synonymy or false synonymy:

- Two or more etymologically synonymous morphemes corresponding to the same concept as in:

English	Greek	Latin
vein	*phléps phlebós* (phleb-, phlebo-)	*vena* (ven-, vene-)

blood vessel	*aggeion* (angi-, angio-)	*vas* (vas-, vasculo-)
breast	*mastós* (mast-, masto-)	*mamma* (mammo-)
mouth	*stoma stómatos* (stom-, stoma-, stomat-)	*os* (or-, oro-)
face	*prosópon* (prosop-, prosopo-)	*facies* (facio-)
eye	*ophthalmós* (ophthalm-, ophthalmo-)	*oculus* (oculo-)
nose	*rhís rhinós* (rhin-)	*nasus* (nas-)
ear	*oûs otós* (ot-, oto-)	*auris* (auri-)
tongue	*glóssa* (gloss-, glossa-)	*lingua* (linguo-)
spine	*rháchis* (rachi-, rachio-)	*spina* (spin-, spino)
white	*leukós* (leuk-, leuko-)	*albus* (alb-, albi-)
milk	*gála gálaktos* (gal-)	*lac lactis* (lac-)
sugar	*glykys* (gluc-, gluco-)	*sácharon* (sacc-)

- The variety of eponyms associated with names of discoverers or inventors where sometimes two, three or more names are associated with the same concept, as in the following example: Basedow's disease, Flajani's disease, Graves' disease, Parry's disease, all of which refer to exophtalmic goitre.

- Equivalent scientific names such as atrophic arthritis, chronic infectious arthritis, proliferative arthritis, and rheumatoid arthritis, in English; or maladie de Heine-Médin, paralysie spinale infantile, and polyomyélite anterieure aigüe, in French.

- The Latin names of nomenclatures such as the *Nomina Anatomica* and the traditional scientific and popular names for the same concepts. Here botanical, zoological and chemical nomenclatures should be included.

- Coexistence of two synonyms due to changes in modern nomenclatures. For example, in chemical nomenclature the traditional term 'phosphoglyceride' has been replaced by 'glycerophospholipid'. For a while both terms will appear in texts, which may cause confusion.

- The doublets of technical names and their popular synonyms in some languages:

Cephalalgia	Headache
Hypertension	High blood pressure
Buccopharingeal	Mouth and throat

Tachycardia	Racing heart
Antithrombotic	Blood clotting treatment
Diuresis	More urine than normal
Haemorrhage	Bleeding

- The different ways of naming the same drug: the international non-proprietary name (World Health Organization), the trade name of each company and the common name in each country. The international non-proprietary name for Nolotil®, one of the most common analgesics in Spain, recommended by the World Health Organization is metamizole. Yet, as pointed out by Navarro (2005: 206), it is rare to find its international non-proprietary name. Instead, we find it named by different common names in different countries: dipyrone if the text comes from UK or USA; analgin if it comes from India, China or Russia; noramidopyrine if it comes from France; noraminophenazone if it comes from Hungary or Yugoslavia; and so on.

- The accepted loans — mainly from English — in cases where there is a term in the other language, as in stress, bypass, feedback, shock, test, borderline, etc.

- Synonyms coming from the common language, such as poison and venom.

- Acronyms — such as AIDS — and the full form of the concepts they designate — Acquired Immunodeficiency Syndrome — are also a type of synonymy that translators should bear in mind.

- Quasi-synonymous terms that have different shades of meaning such as disease, illness, condition, disorder, and sickness.

- False synonyms as in the relationship between a Hypernym (general term) and a hyponym (specific term), as in the general term artery and a very specific kind of artery such as right coronary artery.

- False synonyms due to partial coincidence of meanings as in 'asphyxia' and 'apnoea'; 'trial' and 'study'; 'mortality' and 'lethality'; 'pathology' and 'disease'; 'aetiology' and 'cause'; 'case' and 'patient'; 'dosage' and 'dose'; 'incidence' and 'prevalence'; 'theory' and 'hypothesis'; 'accuracy' and 'precision'; 'follow' and 'observe'; 'gender' and 'sex'; 'vaccinate' and 'immunize'; 'infectious' and 'contagious'.

Polysemy

A polysemous term is a term that has more than one meaning. Here are some examples:

body	body fluids, amyloid body, adrenal body, Golgy body, etc.
bug	bed bug, beet bug, croton bug, flu bug, etc.
case	brain case, case history, case report, etc.
contagion	transmission of infectious disease, infectious disease, cause of infectious disease
growth	cell differentiation, growth hormone, muscular growth, etc.
head	head trauma, head nurse, drum head, etc.
hurt	damage, ache, harm, deteriorate, offend, etc.
leg	lower leg, elephant leg, milk leg, etc.
period	menstruation, period of time
power	electric power, will power, mental powers, power unit, etc.
pressure	atrial pressure, high intracranial pressure, blood pressure, haemostasis by digital presure, etc.
record	birth record, clinical record, resting record, etc.
sense	common sense, body sense, sense of discomfort, etc.
strain	bacterial strain, strained muscle, ventricular strain, etc.
stress	mental stress, biochemical stress, torsional stress, wall stress, etc.
temperature	room temperature, to have a temperature

As happens with synonymy, polysemy can originate in eponyms, and in Greek and Latin roots, prefixes or suffixes – 'cervical' can refer to the neck, to the uterus and to the bladder.

Abbreviations and acronyms are sources of polysemy. According to Navarro (2005: 193), the abbreviation CF can have at least 15 meanings: calibration factor, cancer free, cardiac failure, Caucasian female, chemotactic factor, Chiari-Frommel, chick fibroblast, Christmas factor, citrovorum factor, clotting factor, colony factor, complement fixation, contractile force, coronary flow and cystic fibrosis. The acronym BAL can mean blood alcohol level, broncho-alveolar lavage and British antilewisite. rDNA can mean ribosomal DNA and recombinant DNA. And many more.

Another important consequence of polysemy is that different meanings of the same term in the source language may have different designations in the target language, as in the last example of the list above, where in Spanish there is a separate term for each of the meanings: 'temperatura' and 'fiebre'.

As is normally the case in any type of translation, context is what most reliably guides the translator to the choice of the most appropriate meaning activated in the source text.

Homonymy

Homonymous terms are not as frequent as synonymous and polysemous ones. Homonymy normally derives from the formal coincidence of Greek and Latin roots such as metr- (measure and uterus), cario- (becoming rotten and nucleus), hydr- (sweat and water), eco- (house and echo), brachy- (slow and short), aur- (hearing and gold), acu- (needle and hearing), sex- (sex and six).

False friends

Among the most frequent challenges for the medical translator are false friends, that is terms that have a similar form in the source and target language and which may mislead the translator into thinking that their meaning is the same. False friends differ according to the pair of languages involved. However, there are some that are fairly widespread in many modern languages:

- Abortus does not mean abortion but a foetus that is not viable.
- Constipated does not mean to have a cold but to have difficulty in defecating.
- Disorder does not mean lack of order, but alteration or disease.
- Drug does not only mean illegal drug, but also therapeutic substance.
- Evidence does not mean slight indication that something may be true or false, but proof.
- Labour does not mean work or task, but giving birth to a child.
- Sane does not mean healthy in the general sense, but mentally stable.
- In medical English, the adjective fatal is used to mean mortal, whereas in other languages it can have a different meaning.

Neologisms

Neologisms are new terms used to represent and transmit new concepts. They are the result of what we have referred to as the process of terminologizing new medical knowledge (see section 7.1.). They can be either newly formed words or existing words to which new meanings are attached. In both cases, the words may originate in and be borrowed from another language, and then we can speak of loan terms. Sometimes, the new words are formed from existing components as in plantibodies (plant + bodies), nutraceuticals (nutrition + pharmaceuticals), theranostics (therapy + diagnostics).

Neologisms may also come from existing words used metaphorically. Consider the following examples from Genetics: translation, transcription, RNA editing, proofreading, reading frame, messenger RNA, satellite RNA, microsatellite, minisatellite, nested genes, and so on.

Nowadays, most research journals in the biomedical fields are published in English, the *lingua franca* of biomedical research of scientific and technical communication in general. Therefore, most neologisms originate in English and are then translated into a wide range of languages.

When coming across a neologism, medical translators have two types of challenge. On the one hand, understanding the meaning of the English term in the source text. On the other, finding an equivalent term in the target language. Ideally, each language should have an official body responsible for dealing with the translation of neologisms quickly which would save the translator much time and effort.

Nowadays, however, communication in the biomedical fields is very rapid and translators are often required to deal either with the lack of terms in the target language or with the proliferation of alternatives for the same neologism due to the lack of terminological planning and control. Hence, the need for translators to base their decisions on sound criteria that can be applied to any neologism.

According to *Termcat* (Catalan terminological centre), there are three types of criteria: linguistic, terminological and social.

Linguistic criteria

- Ease of pronunciation.
- Spelling conforming to the general rules of the language.
- Correct morphology (formation of plural, derivation, conjugation, etc.).
- Semantic transparency so that the new term represents the concept in a clear and accurate way.
- Syntactic flexibility of the new term so that it can be used in any sentence and any context.

Terminological criteria

- Avoidance of ambiguity and homonymy.
- Harmonious integration of the term in the network of concepts and forms to which it belongs.
- Formal analogy with semantically related terms within the same language.
- Formal analogy with the same term in other languages so as to facilitate internationalization.
- Conformity with the recommendations of international standardization

bodies.
- Preference for Greek or Latin forms whenever possible.
- Consensus among field specialists.

Social criteria

- Real need for a neologism.
- Consideration of the profile of the user.
- Social and professional prestige of the word.
- Avoidance of snobbery.
- Avoidance of pejorative, sexist or racist connotations.
- Brevity and simplicity so that it can be easily used.
- Memorability.
- Possibilities of spreading and becoming broadly accepted and used.

Updating of nomenclatures

Even nomenclatures are not completely fixed entities. In fact, this would be impossible, since research is constantly modifying the state of knowledge in all disciplines. For instance, the following bacteria have been renamed recently: *Campylobacter pyloridis* has become *Helicobacter pyroli*; *Salmonella paratyphi* is now called *Salmonella enteritidis*. And likewise many more bacteria, viruses, names of diseases, etc. However, some nomenclatures vary more than others. For example, the international names of diseases and the international names of drugs are more variable than the international names used in Botany or Zoology.

The translator's position vis a vis terminological variation

When we are faced with terminological variation we realize that often there are no *a priori* solutions awaiting us in monolingual or bilingual dictionaries. Rather, there are *ad hoc* solutions for each text and for each assignment that we discover through common sense, reasoning, and the study of parallel texts.

A frequent and challenging phenomenon in medical translation arises from the fact that synonyms do not coincide in different languages. We might find a variety of synonyms in the target language where there is only one term in the source language, and vice-versa. Take, for instance, the term 'stem cells' in English and the range of possibilities in other languages, such as Spanish: 'células precursoras', 'células troncales', 'células primordiales', 'citoblastos', 'células madre', 'células pluripotenciales', and so on. Searching the web or specialized databases for the frequency of use of the various synonyms can help us decide which of them to choose. Other criteria we must bear in mind are the type of task we have been assigned by the client, the reader's profile, and the fact that terminological choices may depend on the genre of the target text.

When translating medical texts we find a whole range of terminological phenomena: from completely internationalized nomenclatures to popular terms, to de-terminologized concepts. Different strategies and skills are required to translate them.

On the right in Fig. 7.4 terms are used to allow communication between experts and depend more on the internal organization of the discipline. They are used internationally. As a consequence, they are less culturally marked and more neutral. At this extreme of the spectrum, equivalence is of a more static nature and the task of the translator is less creative.

De-terminolo-gized concepts An infection of the nails caused by a fungus	*Popular terms* Nail fungus infection	*Traditional scientific term* Onychomycosis	*Nomenclatures* Tinea unguium
← ·· →			
+ Text-bound + Layman communication + Localized + Varied + Culturally marked + Dynamic equivalence		+ Discipline-bound + Expert-to-expert communication + Internationalized + Standardized + Neutral + Static equivalence	

Figure 7.4. Ways of expressing specialized concepts

Moving to the left in the same figure, we see that terms are used to allow communication between experts and non-experts, and also between non-experts. Terms are more culturally marked, there is more diversity of denominations within one language and between different languages, and terms are more text and context bound. Therefore, the notion of equivalence becomes more dynamic.

Terminological variation demands both caution and creativity from the translator. On the one hand, translators must watch out for possible asymmetries and divergences within and between languages. On the other, they must be ready to bridge the gap of variations in cases where they are required to provide solutions for neologisms that have not yet become established.

7.5 De-terminologizing the text

> Homer, I'm afraid you'll have to undergo a coronary bypass operation.
> *Say it in English, Doc.* You're going to need open-heart surgery.
> *Spare me your medical mumbo-jumbo. Could you dumb it down a shade?*
> We're going to cut you open and tinker with your ticker.
>
> (Matt Groening, The Simpsons)

Traditionally scientific and technical translation training has focused on terms in the source text and their equivalents in the target language. And indeed translators often invest a considerable amount of their time searching for terminological equivalents in the target language. Substituting the terms of one language for those of another language, however, is not the only task medical translators have to deal with as far as terminology is concerned. Sometimes more complex operations are required.

As we saw at the beginning of the chapter, terminologizing is the process whereby concepts are established and specific words are attached to them in order to represent and communicate them. The result is medical terms, units of specialized knowledge meant to facilitate the organization and transmission of medical knowledge mainly in specialized contexts, such as research, clinical practice, and higher education. When the context of communication of medical knowledge moves from the specialists in the source language to the general public in the target language, then new communication needs arise.

Imagine the following assignment. You are given a research article in English and are asked to produce a press release in the target language to be distributed to the general public through the mass media, or an abridged version for patients. As well as selecting the most important information for your summary, you will have to deal with terms so that a non-specialist reader can understand them. In some cases you may give a definition of the concept and then introduce the term. In some other cases you may choose to use a popular version of the same term. This we call "de-terminologization". This is quite a mouthful, but you may never need to use it. What is important is that you recognize the concept underlying it.

For the specialist, terms and other units of specialized knowledge (USK) are a quick, clear, precise, way of transmitting information. For the man in the street, the same terms hinder communication. Agencies specializing in medical translation often focus on this aspect. Here is a typical advertisement for such services:

Patient information
Medical translation written for your patients. Our specialists translate for your audience's culture and education level, for accuracy and ease of comprehension.

De-terminologizing the text may be a requirement of the assignment, especially in translations that need to be adapted extensively. This can be done in four ways. Depending on the assignment, one or more of the following procedures will be used:

- Scientific terms are kept and followed by explanations.

Example of source text: Most **dyskinesias** are due to basal ganglia disorders, although precise neuroanatomic correlates are usually lacking. The various dyskinesias form a continuum from the lightning-like flickers of myoclonus to the slow, writhing patterns of **dystonia**.

Example of gloss in the target language: Most **dyskinesias** (impairment of voluntary movements resulting in fragmented or jerky motions) are due to basal ganglia disorders, although precise neuroanatomic correlates are usually lacking. The various dyskinesias form a continuum from the lightning-like flickers of myoclonus to the slow, writhing patterns of **dystonia** (abnormal tonicity of muscle, characterized by prolonged, repetitive muscle contractions that may cause twisting or jerking movements of the body or a body part.)

- Scientific terms are kept in brackets after the explanations.

Example of source text: Usually, the hands, arms, and legs are most affected, in that order. Jaw, tongue, forehead, and eyelids may also be affected, but the voice escapes the tremor. In many patients, only rigidity occurs; tremor is absent. Rigidity progresses, and **bradykinesia, hypokinesia,** and **akinesia** appear.

Example of gloss in the target language: Usually, the hands, arms, and legs are most affected, in that order. Jaw, tongue, forehead, and eyelids may also be affected, but the voice escapes the tremor. In many patients, only rigidity occurs; tremor is absent. Rigidity progresses, and movement becomes slow (**brady-kinesia**), decreased (**hypokinesia**), and difficult to initiate (**akinesia**).

- Scientific terms are replaced by popular terms.

Example: Symptoms typically begin abruptly with headache, followed by steadily increasing neurologic deficits. Large **haemorrhages**, when located in the hemispheres, produces **hemiparesis**.

Example of gloss in the target language: Symptoms typically begin abruptly with headache, followed by steadily increasing neurologic deficits. Intense bleeding, when located in the hemispheres, produces paralysis on one side of the body.

- Scientific terms are completely avoided and replaced by explanations.

Example of source text: Most **dyskinesias** are due to basal ganglia disorders, although precise neuroanatomic correlates are usually lacking. The various dyskinesias form a continuum from the lightning-like flickers of myoclonus to the slow, writing patterns of **dystonia**.

Example of gloss in the target language: Most impairment of voluntary movements is due to basal ganglia disorders, although precise neuroanatomic correlates are usually lacking. The various dyskinesias form a continuum from the lightning-like flickers of myoclonus to the slow, writing patterns of abnormal tonicity of muscle.

According to the assignment and the language combination, you will use one of the above procedures or a combination of them.

De-terminologizing the terms in the sense of paraphrasing them *viva voce* in the reading and understanding process may also help to improve comprehension of the source text before producing the target text.

Task 5. De-terminologizing a text addressed to the general public.

The following sentences have been taken from a manual for physicians. Translate them into your target language taking into account that your target readership is the general public. Pay special attention to the way you present the technical terms in bold type. Do your best to make your reader understand them adequately.

Colonic inertia occurs in elderly or invalid patients, especially if bedridden. The colon does not respond to the usual stimuli that promote evacuation, or accessory stimuli normally provided by eating and physical activity are lacking.

Arrhythmias that cause **hemodynamic upset** are usually sustained **bradycardias** or **tachycardias** and may be life threatening.

A comprehensive **ophthalmic** examination is essential for diagnosis and prompt treatment. Examination includes visualization of the angle by **gonioscopy**, **IOP (normal intraocular pressure)** measurement, visual field examination and, most importantly, examination of the **optic disks**.

7.6 Further tasks

Task 6. Comparing and evaluating definitions of the same term

Read definitions of the same medical terms in different dictionaries and decide which of them is more useful to you for your particular translation purposes.

Task 7. Paraphrasing the meaning of terms

Paraphrase the meaning of terms of Greek and Latin origin according to their etymological form. Use the information provided in the tables in Appendix 2.

Task 8. Forming terms

Using the tables in Appendix 2, form terms with one Greek or Latin root and with different Greek or Latin prefixes and suffixes. Check whether they exist and, if so, what they mean.

Task 9. Comparing and evaluating definitions of the same term

1) Look for the traditional scientific terms in your language for anatomical, botanical and zoological terms in Latin.
2) Look for the popular terms in your language for anatomical, botanical and zoological terms in Latin.
3) Look for the nomenclatures of popular and traditional scientific terms in your language.

Task 10. Names of drugs

1) Choose some commercial drugs in your country and look for their non-proprietary names.
2) Find a drug that has different commercial names in different countries.

7.7 Further reading

Casselman, W. (1998) *A Dictionary of Medical Derivations. The Real Meaning of Medical Terms*, London and New York: Parthenon Publishing Group.
Dunmore, C.W. and R.M. Fleischer (2004) *Medical Terminology. Excercises in Etymology*, Philadelphia: F.A. Davies. 3rd edition

English Centre of the University of Hong Kong (2004) *Medical Terminology*, <http://ec.hku.hk/mt>.

Gutiérrez Roda, B. (1998) *La ciencia empieza en la palabra. Análisis e historia del lenguaje científico,* Barcelona: Península.

Halliday, M.A.K. (1998) 'Things and relations: Rematicising experience as technical knowledge', in J.R. Martin and R. Veel (eds) *Reading Science. Critical and Functional Perspectives of Discourses of Science*, London and New York: Routledge, 185-235.

Haubrich, W.S. (2003) *Medical Meanings. A Glossary of Word Origins*, Philadelphia: American College of Physicians, 2nd edition.

Lafleur-Brooks, M. (2002) *Exploring Medical Language. A Student-Directed Approach*, St. Louis: Mosby Inc., 5th edition.

"Montalt, Vicent (2005) *Manual de traducció cientificotècnica*, in Biblioteca de Traducció i Interpretació, Vic: Eumo.".

Navarro, F. (2005) *Diccionario crítico de dudas inglés-español de dudas de medicina,* Madrid: McGraw-Hill.

Quérin, Serge (2001) 'Emploi de termes hybrides gréco-latins dans le langage médical', *Meta* 46(1): 7-15.

Steiner, S.S. (2002) *Quick Medical Terminology: A Self-Teaching Guide*, Indianapolis: John Wiley and Sons.

Appendix 1. Translation problems: strategies, procedures and solutions

MAIN CONCEPT	POTENTIAL PROBLEMS TO BE SOLVED	TRANSLATION STRATEGIES: STEPS TO ACCESS ACCEPTABLE PROCEDURES	TRANSLATION PROCEDURES: POTENTIAL FINAL SOLUTIONS
General guidelines	Basic strategies valid for most translation problems. First steps that should always be followed.	aim at understanding globally as much as possible: anatomy, histology, physiology, pharmacology, etc., but not necessarily at the same level as a medical specialist. Learn when to stop! contact directly with the clients or authors for photographs, feedback on obscure or invented terms, phraseology, etc. consult fellow translators, linguists and medical specialists (also, online groups), obtain the references in the bibliography of the text you have to translate, put the translation draft aside for a few hours and return to read the target text later, so that the possible interfering influence of the source text patterning is reduced, read, watch TV, listen to the radio, surf the Internet, visit source and target language countries frequently, use dictionaries in the target language *or in languages related to it* (beware of false friends).	see under each heading.

Abbreviations and acronyms (mainly chapter 7)	coined by the author,	ask medical specialists,	coin a translation the first time it appears in the text,
	see below: *eponyms, neologisms, no equivalent and resourcing,*	contact author or client,	see *eponyms, neologisms, no equivalent and resourcing,*
	standard acronyms and abbreviations,	intratextual referencing: scan the whole text carefully in case it is explained further on,	show the client parallel texts, write it in the source language and between brackets, e.g. "source language word (SLW)", and then paraphrase it.
	the author leaves them in the source language with no explanation,	look at the beginning of text or the first time the acronym or abbreviation appears,	
	the author leaves the acronym or abbreviation in the source language, but refers to the concept in the target language,	look for specific publications on the topic: parallel texts,	
	the author translates them according to the his or her own criteria, explaining it or not,	see *eponyms, neologisms, no equivalent and resourcing.*	
	the author uses what Jammal (1999: 227) calls "siglomanie", that is, an overuse of abbreviations and acronyms, without explaining the meaning of the letters,		
	the author alternates them in both languages (especially in oral translations),		
	the client prefers the translator to use the English version in spite of there existing an equivalent in the other language,		
	the same abbreviation is used for several concepts.		

Cohesion and coherence (mainly chapter 4)			
absence of an element in the sentence,	analyze target language parallel texts on the same subject and corresponding to the same text type,	adding,	
ambiguity,		deleting,	
change of meaning according to word order,	be aware of target language legibility and text conventions,	explicitation,	
dangling participles,	logical and lateral thinking,	rechunking (reorganizing or renumbering)	
deictics,	change of word order ("puzzle" with words and clauses until they "fit"),	reordering,	
false comparatives,		repunctuating,	
gender,	content chunking (discovering the internal structure of a text with the help of wh-questions)	see *phraseology* and *resourcing*,	
genre,		translate titles at the very end.	
passive / active voice,	semantic chunking: up, down or sideways,		
person / number,	prepare a gap-filling text for another reader to discuss different translation options (paragraphs, sentences), producing different lexical chains,		
restrictions of word order,			
see *phraseology* and *resourcing*,	READ: aloud, to somebody else, by somebody else, focus on intonation, see *phraseology* and *resourcing*,		
syntactic calques,			
syntactic juxtaposition: a number of adjectives can follow one another, or an adjective precedes two nouns,	translate after having read the whole paragraph: *understanding* must be foremost, next to *knowing*.		
text type,			
verb tense.			

Collocations (mainly chapters 3 and 4)	affixes, culture-specific collocations, different collocation in source and target languages, engrossing effect of source text patterning can lead, e.g., to involuntary calques, marked collocations in the source text, misinterpreting the meaning of source language collocation, spelling (often similar, but not identical), tension between accuracy and naturalness, word order.	be alerted to the potential influence of the source text, consult specific references for collocations in source and target languages, consult parallel texts, consult a specialist, evaluate the significance of a potential change in meaning, read aloud to somebody else.	paraphrase, reword or change word order as appropriate in target language, translation by a neutral word, translation by a collocation, translation by a marked collocation depending on the constraints of the target language and the purpose of the translation.
Cultural references (mainly chapter 5)	different modes of expression: linguistic and extralinguistic, different world references.	contact source and target language communities, from physicians to patients, journals, etc. observe, understand and adapt to different approaches to Speech Acts, Grice's Maxims, Politeness rules, etc. in both communities, read publications on the topic and on community interpreting, understand and adapt to high and low context cultures.	apply translation procedures related to the translation of cultural references (see chapter 3): exoticism, cultural borrowing, calque, transliteration, communicative translation, cultural transplantation, cultural chunking: up, down and sideways, paraphrasing, translation by addition, translation by deleting, translation by illustration.

Eponyms (mainly chapter 7)	an eponym in the source language corresponds to a descriptive word or expression in the target language or vice versa,	see *abbreviations and acronyms, neologisms, no equivalence* and *resourcing.*	see *abbreviations and acronyms, neologisms, no equivalence* and *resourcing.*
	false friend eponyms,		
	see *abbreviations and acronyms, neologisms, no equivalence* and *resourcing,*		
	the proper name in the source language is a common name in the target language or vice versa,		
	the same illness may have different eponyms or names,		
	there may be an eponym for the same concept, but a different one,		
	there may exist an eponym in one language, but not in the other.		
False friends and reversed terms (above all, affixes) (mainly chapter 7)	a word looks or sounds the same in the source and target languages, but has a different meaning,	consult false friends articles and dictionaries, if available in your language combination,	see *No equivalent,*
	see *No equivalent.*	see *No equivalent,*	use the appropriate word or paraphrase.
		set up your own glossary of false friends and affixes.	

Idioms and metaphors (mainly chapter 5)	see *cultural references* and *resourcing*.	
difference between the convention, context and frequency of use in the source and target languages,		coin an idiom following target language conventions,
false friends,		see *cultural references* and *resourcing*,
idiom used in the source text both in its literal and idiomatic sense at the same time,		translation by an idiom or metaphor of similar meaning and form,
no equivalent in the target language,		translation by an idiom or metaphor of similar meaning but differing form,
partial correspondence: same meaning, different metaphors, idioms, cultural references,		paraphrasing,
partial correspondence: polysemy - not all the meanings of the expression can be translated,		omission,
partial correspondence: same meaning, but different lexical or syntactic construction,		compensation,
see *cultural references* and *resourcing*, similar counterpart in the target language with a different context of use.		rewording,
		translation by paraphrase using unrelated words,
		translation by illustration.

Category	Problem	Resourcing	Strategy
Neologisms (mainly chapter 7)	the author coins a new word or expression, a new notion is expressed in a term that is not yet in the dictionary, loan words in the source text, see *abbreviations and acronyms* and *eponyms, no equivalent* and *resourcing*.	see *abbreviations and acronyms* and *eponyms, no equivalent* and *resourcing*.	see *abbreviations and acronyms, eponyms, no equivalent* and *resourcing*, coin new words by following the word formation and medical language norms in the target language and put the source language word between brackets (*SLW*) the first time it appears in the text, coin new words by looking at dictionary prefaces and the principles they follow to accept or reject terms.
No equivalent (mainly chapter 7)	cultural references differences in expressive meaning, differences in form, differences in frequency and purpose of using specific forms, differences in physical or interpersonal perspective, idioms, in dictionary, but does not seem to fit text,	consult a specialist, look in monolingual dictionary: source language, target language and related languages, look in bilingual and specialized dictionaries: source language, target language and related languages, look in medical encyclopedias: source language, target language and related languages, parallel texts: look for similar contexts, see *abbreviations and acronyms, eponyms, neologisms and resourcing*.	explicitation, footnote, see *abbreviations and acronyms, eponyms, neologisms and resourcing*, translation by a more general word (superordinate), translation by a more neutral/less expressive word, translation by cultural substitution, translation by illustration, translation by omission,

	Problems	Strategies
	more than one translation may be possible, not in the dictionary, see *abbreviations and acronyms, eponyms, neologisms and resourcing*, the source and target languages make different distinctions in meaning, the source language concept is not lexicalized in the target language, the source language word is semantically complex, the target language lacks a specific term (hyponym), the target language lacks a superordinate.	translation by paraphrase using a related word, translation by paraphrase using unrelated words, translation using a loan word or loan word plus explanation, transliteration.
Phraseology (mainly chapter 4)	depends on country of origin, if English is the target language, because of the status of English as *lingua franca* (culture influences style, syntactic relaying, etc),	class drilling written exercises for awareness, create a personal (online) dictionary of sentence correspondences, read a lot about the topic so that it is partly acquired by "osmosis", adapt to target language norms and conventions.

			see *abbreviations and acronyms, eponyms, neologisms* and *no equivalent,*
	depends on text type and on the part of the text being translated, phraseology also of statistics and technical fields.	role plays – adapt oral language and reinforce vocabulary and speech acts, text editing activities (self, peer and team editing), translator workbenches, memory, etc (software), underline parallel texts.	
Resourcing (mainly chapter 6)	definitions not listed in order of frequency, dictionaries: not totally updated (even Internet), inadequate translations: direct equivalences from source language, lack of different registers in translations, many translations of the same term, no different linguistic varieties, no grammar information,	be careful with medical terms defined in general dictionaries, check year, author and place of publication, check register, origin, pronunciation if necessary, synonyms if any, etc. consult a specialist, consult paper and online dictionaries, consult updated medical web sites, extratextual resourcing (reference works and experts),	

			see abbreviations and acronyms, collocations, cultural references, eponyms, false friends, idioms and metaphors, neologisms, no equivalent, resourcing.
	no (or few) example sentences, no contrasted charts or tables (weights, etc.) no diagrams or pictures, see *abbreviations and acronyms, eponyms, neologisms* and *no equivalent,* translations do not exist, translations do not seem appropriate.	intratextual resourcing (in the same document, there is sometimes a solution), look at dictionaries of related fields, look at dictionaries of related languages, look at Latin and Greek dictionaries, look up new words in new editions of dictionaries, parallel texts, but never only one, see *abbreviations and acronyms, eponyms, neologisms* and *no equivalent,* sequence the search appropriately: monolingual (source language) - bilingual – monolingual (target language) - Latin or Greek – parallel texts – experts, use encyclopedias with illustrations, use new generation dictionaries on calques, false friends, etc. Word Finders or Reversicons.	
Terminology (mainly chapter 7)	abbreviations and acronyms, collocations, evolution of medical terms: e.g. archaic words,	activities related to chunking words, becoming familiar with Latin and Greek affixes,	

eponyms,	guess through the context, but always check in a monolingual dictionary or with a specialist,
erratic creation of medical terms,	
false friends,	learn / revise basic school Biology, Chemistry, Natural Sciences…,
idioms and metaphors,	
Latin and Greek affixes and word combination,	look up words and expressions by means of their synonyms,
lay terms vs. medical terms,	
neologisms,	*see abbreviations and acronyms, collocations, cultural references, eponyms, false friends, idioms and metaphors, neologisms, no equivalent, resourcing.*
no equivalent,	
proliferation of synonyms,	
same word can have different meaning according to context,	
see abbreviations and acronyms, collocations, cultural references, eponyms, false friends, idioms and metaphors, neologisms, no equivalent, resourcing,	
terms determined by geography or by cultural preferences,	
word combination rules.	

Appendix 2. Latin and Greek roots for medical terminology

Since the following information is not presented in alphabetical order or in an exhaustive way, it is of little use when trying to find out the meaning of a particular Greek or Latin term found in a text in the process of translating. For that purpose, you should use an etymological dictionary. The information presented in this section is conceived of mainly as material for self-study and as a starting point for the University teacher.

Some of the most common terms have been grouped thematically: first, general concepts about health and disease, then, the parts of the body: mouth, head, trunk, and limbs; the cardiovascular system; and the urinary and reproductive systems. Finally etymological information relating to: substances; position of objects or processes in space and time; quality of things; quantity of things; light and colour; shapes; and frequent actions.

The first column indicates the general concept, part of the body, substance, position, quality, quantity, colour, shape or action in English. The second column contains the root, prefix or suffix on which the term is based. The third column gives the meaning of each root, prefix or suffix. Finally, in the fourth column examples are provided of each of the root, prefix or suffix.

General concepts about health and disease	Root, prefix, suffix	Meaning	Examples of terms
Birth (G. tókos)	Toco-	Denoting childbirth.	Tocography
Life (G. bíos)	Bio-	Denoting life.	Biopsy
Life (L. vivus)	Vivi-	Denoting life, alive.	Viviparity
Body (G. sôma, sômatos)	Somat- Somato- -soma	Denoting the body.	Somatoagnosis
Mind, heart. (G. thymos)	-thymia	Denoting mind, and heart, as the seat of strong feelings or passion.	Cyclothymia

Diaphragm, mind, heart. (G. phrén)	-phrenia	Denoting diaphragm, mind, and heart, as the seat of emotions.	Schizophrenia
Death (G. thánatos)	Thanato-	Denoting death.	Thanatomania
Cell (G. kytos, meaning a hollow)	Cyt- Cyto-	Combining forms meaning cell.	Cytokinesis
Immature precursor cell (G. blastós, meaning germ)	Blasto- -blast	Indicating an immature precursor cell of the type indicated by the preceding word in the case of the suffix.	Lymphoblast
Tissue (G. histiós)	Histio- Histo-	Relating to tissue.	Histological anatomy
Gland (G. adén)	Aden- Adeno-	Denoting relation to a gland.	Adenotomy
Abnormal condition	-osis	Suffix meaning a process, condition or state, usually abnormal or diseased.	Necrosis
Inflammation	-itis	Suffix denoting inflammation.	Dermatitis
Morbid condition	-iasis	Suffix denoting a condition or state, particularly morbid.	Strongyloidiasis
Disease (G. nósos)	Noso-	Combining form relating to disease.	Nosology

Pain (G. álgos)	Alge- Algesi- Algio- Algo- -algia	Combining forms meaning pain.	Analgesic
Pain (G. odyne)	Odyn- Odyno-	Combining forms meaning pain.	Odynophagia
Stroke (G. plegé)	-plegia	Suffix denoting paralysis.	Hemiplegia
Cancer (G. karkínos, meaning crab)	Carcin- Carcino-	Relating to cancer.	Carcinoma
Mass, lump (G. ónkos)	Onco-	Denoting a tumour or some relation to a tumour.	Oncogenesis
Tumour (G.-oma)	-oma	Suffix denoting a tumour or neoplasm.	Atheroma
Wound (G. traûma)	Traum- Traumat- Traumato-	Combining forms denoting wound, injury.	Traumatology
Nourishment (G. trophé)	Troph- Tropho- -trophy -trophic	Combining forms meaning food, nutrition.	Atrophoderma Hypotrophy

Parts of the body I: mouth, head, trunk and limbs	*Root, prefix, suffix*	*Meaning*	*Examples of terms*
Head (G. kephalé)	Cephal- Cephalo-	Denoting the head.	Cephalalgia
Brain (L. enképhalos)	Encephalo-	Indicating the brain or some relationship thereto.	Encephalitis

Nerve (G. neûron)	Neur- Neuri- Neuro-	Combining forms denoting a nerve or relating to the nervous system.	Neurolepsis
Skull (G. kraníon)	Crani- Cranio-	Denoting the skull.	Craniotomy
Face (G. prósopon)	Prosop- Prosopo-	Denoting the face.	Prosopalgia
Face (L. facies)	Facio-	Denoting the face.	Facioplegia
Eye (G. ophthalmós)	Ophthalm- Ophthalmo-	Denoting relationship to the eye.	Ophthalmomalacia
Eye (G. óps)	-opia	Suffix meaning vision.	Myopia
Eye (L. oculus)	Oculo-	Denoting the eye.	Oculomotor nerve
Nose (G. rhís rhinós)	Rhin-	Denoting the nose.	Rhinitis
Nose (L. nasus)	Nas-	Denoting the nose.	Nasal cavity
Ear (G. oûs otós)	Ot- Oto-	Denoting the ear.	Otolaryngology
Ear (L. auris)	Auri-	Denoting the ear.	Auriscope
Mouth (L. bucca)	Bucco-	Relating to the mouth and the cheek.	Buccal mucosa
Mouth (G. stoma stómatos)	Stom- Stomat- Stomato-	Relating to the mouth.	Stomatitis
Mouth (L. os oris)	Or- Oro-	Relating to the mouth.	Oral herpes
Gingiva (L. gingiva)	Gingivo-	Relating to the gingivae.	Gingivostomatitis

Jaw (G. gnáthos)	Gnath- Gnatho-	Combining forms relating to the jaw.	Gnathostomiasis
Lip (G. cheîlos)	Cheil- Cheilo-	Denoting relationship to the lips.	Cheilotomy
Lip (L. labium)	Labio-	Denoting relationship to the lips.	Labial teeth
Tongue (G. glôssa)	Gloss- Glosso-	Combining forms relating to the tongue.	Glossoplegia
Tongue (L. lingua)	Lingu- Linguo-	Denoting the tongue.	Lingual bone
Tooth (L. dens dentis)	Dent- Denti- Dento-	Combining forms relating to the teeth.	Dentalgia
Neck (G. tráchelos)	Trachel- Trachelo-	Combining forms denoting neck.	Trachelocele
Neck (L. cervix cervicis)	Cervico-	Relating to a cervix, or neck, in any sense.	Cervical osteoarthritis
Chest (G. stéthos)	Steth- Stetho-	Denoting the chest.	Stethoparalysis
Chest (G. thorax thorakos)	Thoraco-	Denoting the chest.	Thoracopathy
Lung (G. pneúmon, pneumonos)	Pneumo- Pneumon- Pneumono-	Denoting the lungs, air or gas, or respiration.	Pneumonia
Breast (G. mastós)	Mast- Masto-	Denoting the breast.	Mastalgia
Breast (L. mamma)	Mammo-	Denoting the breast.	Mammography
Breast (G. mazos)	Mazo-	Combining form relating to the breast.	Mazopathy

Rib (G. pleurá, meaning side)	Pleuro-	Denoting the ribs.	Pleuropneumonia
Rib (L. costa)	Costo-	Relating to the ribs.	Costovertebral angle
Abdomen (G. lapára)	Laparo-	Denoting the loins or, less properly, the abdomen in general.	Laparocele
Abdomen (L. abdomen abdominis)	Abdomino-	Relating to the abdomen	Abdominoscopy
Extremity (G. ákros)	Acro-	Extremity, tip, end, peak, topmost.	Acromegaly
Shoulder (G. ómos)	Omo-	Indicating relationship to the shoulder.	Omoclavicular trigone
Arm (L. bracchium)	Brachi- Brachio-	Denoting relationship to the arm.	Brachiocephalic
Elbow (L. cubitum)	Cubit- Cubito-	Denoting the elbow.	Median cubital vein
Hand (L. cheír cheirós)	Quir- Quiro-	Denoting the hand.	Chiroplasty
Finger (G. dáktylos)	Dactyl- Dactylo-	Relating to the fingers, and sometimes to the toes.	Dactylographer
Finger (L. digitus)	Digit-	Denoting the fingers.	Digital rectal examination
Hip (L. coxa)	Cox-	Denoting the hip.	Coxalgia
Knee (G. góny)	Gon Goni-	Denoting the knee.	Gonococcal arthritis
Knee (L. genu)	Genu-	Denoting the knee	Genuflexion

Foot (G. poús, podós)	Pod- Podo-	Indicating foot or foot-shaped.	Podalgia
Bone (G. ostéon)	Ost- Oste- Osteo-	Denoting bone.	Osteocarcinoma
Marrow (G. myelós)	Myel- Myelo-	Denoting the bone marrow, the spinal cord and medulla oblonga, and the myelin sheath of nerve fibres.	Myelogram
Joint (G. árthron)	Arthr- Arthro-	Denoting a joint or articulation.	Arthritis
Spine (G. rháchis)	Rachi- Rachio-	Denoting the spine.	Rachitis
Spine (L. spina)	Spin- Spino-	Denoting the spine.	Spinal fluid
Vertebra (G. spóndylos)	Spondyl- Spondylos-	Combining forms denoting the vertebrae.	Spondylitis
Bowels (G. énteron)	Enter- Entero-	Relating to the intestines.	Enteric infection
Anus (G. proktós)	Proct- Proctos-	Combining forms denoting anus.	Proctoscopy
Spleen (G. splén)	Splen- Spleno-	Denoting the spleen.	Splenial gyrus
Skin (G. dermas dérmatos)	Derm- Derma- Dermat- Dermato- Dermo-	Combining forms signifying skin.	Dermatophytosis

Parts of the body II: cardiovascular system	Root, prefix, suffix	Meaning	Examples of terms
Heart (G. kardía)	Cardi- Cardio- -cardia	Combining forms denoting the heart.	Cardiogram
Blood (G. haîma haímatos)	Haem- Haema- Haemat- Haemato- Haemo-	Combining forms meaning blood.	Haemophilic
Blood clot (G. thrómbos)	Thromb- Thrombo-	Combining forms denoting blood clot or relation thereto.	Thrombolysis
Blood vessel (G. aggeion, meaning vas)	Angi- Angio-	Relating to blood or lymph vessels.	Angioma
Blood vessel (L. vas)	Vas- Vasculo- Vaso-	Denotating a blood vessel.	Vasoconstriction
Vein (G. phléps, phlebós)	Phleb- Phlebo-	Combining form denoting vein.	Phlebitis
Vein (L. vena)	Ven- Vene-	Denotating the veins.	Venectomy
Dilated vein (L. varix varicis)	Varico-	Denotating a varix or varicosity.	Varicocele

Parts of the body III: urinary and reproductive systems	Root, prefix, suffix	Meaning	Examples of terms
Kidney (G. nephrós)	Nephr- Nephro-	Combining forms denoting the kidney.	Nephritis

Bladder (G. kystis kystidos)	Cyst- Cysti- Cysto-	Combining forms relating to the bladder.	Cystectomy
Urine (G. oûron)	Ure- Ureo-	Combining forms relating to urine.	Ureagenesis
Ovary (G. oón meaning egg and phorós meaning that carries or produces)	Oophor- Oophoro-	Combining forms denoting the ovary.	Oophoralgia
Womb (G. hystéra)	Hyster- Hystero-	Combining forms meaning womb.	Hysterography
Womb (G. metra)	Metr- Metra- Metro-	Combining form denoting the uterus.	Metritis
Penis (G. phallós)	Phall- Phalli- Phallo-	Denoting the penis.	Phallodynia
Vagina (G. kólpos)	Colp- Colpo-	Denoting the vagina.	Colpectomy

Substances	*Root, prefix, suffix*	*Meaning*	*Examples of terms*
Something formed (G. plásma)	Plasma- Plasmat- Plasmato- Plasmo-	Denoting plasma.	Plasmablast
Gruel (G. athéré)	Ather- Athero-	Relating to the deposit of gruel-like, soft, pasty materials.	Atherosclerosis

Grit, gristle, cartilage. (G. chóndros)	Chondri- Chondro-	Denoting granular or gritty substance; cartilage or cartilaginous.	Chondrification
Water (G. hydor)	Hydr- Hydro-	Denoting water or association with water.	Hydrophobia
Spring water (G. lympha)	Lymph- Lympho-	Combining forms relating to lymph.	Lymphoma
Milk (G. gála gálaktos)	Galact- Galacto-	Combining forms indicating milk.	Galactopoiesis
Milk (L. lac lactis)	Lact- Lacti- Lacto-	Combining forms indicating milk.	Lactation
Honey (G. mel mellis)	Meli-	Combining form relating to honey or sugar.	Melituria
Sugar (G. glykys)	Glyco-	Denoting relationship to sugars or to glycine.	Glycogen
Sugar (G. sácharon)	Sacch-	Denoting relationship to sugar.	Saccharin
Starch (G. ámylon)	Amylo-	Indicating starch, or polysaccharide nature or origin.	Amylosynthesis
Suet, tallow (L. sebum)	Seb- Sebi- Sebo-	Denoting sebum, sebaceous.	Seborrhoea
Fat (G. lipós)	Lip- Lipo-	Denoting fat.	Lipidosis

Fat (L. adeps)	Adip- Adipo-	Combining forms relating to fat.	Adiposity
Flesh (G. sárx sarkós)	Sarco-	Denoting muscular substance or a resemblance to flesh.	Sarcoma
Stone (G. líthos)	Lith- Litho-	Combining forms relating to a stone or calculus.	Lithodialysis
Potassium (L. kalium)	Kal- Kali-	Denoting potassium.	Kalemia
Glue (G. glia)	Glio-	Combining form meaning glue or gluelike.	Glioblast
Dung (G. kópros)	Copro-	Denoting filth or dung, usually used in referring to faeces.	Coprophagy
Excrement (G. skór)	Scato-	Denoting faeces.	Scatology
Bile (L. bilis)	Bili-	Combining form relating to bile.	Bilirubin
Mucus (G. myxa)	Myx- Myxo-	Combining forms relating to mucus.	Myxopoiesis
Mucus (L. mucus)	Muco-	Combining form for mucus, mucous, mucosa.	Mucous membrane
Pus (G. pyon)	Pyo-	Denoting suppuration or an accumulation of pus.	Pyogenic arthritis

| Wood (G. xylon) | Xyl- Xylo- | Combining forms relating to wood. | Xylose |
| Coal (G. ánthrax ánthrakos) | Anthra- | Denoting coal. | Anthrax |

Position in space or time	Root, prefix, suffix	Meaning	Examples of terms
Place (G. tópos)	Top- Topo-	Denoting place.	Topoanesthesia
Upon (G. epí)	Epi- Epio-	Denoting upon.	Epidermis
Below (L. infra)	Infra-	Denoting a position below the part denoted by the word to which it is joined.	Infraoccipital nerve
Before (L. ante)	Ante-	Denoting before either in time or in space.	Anteflexion
Against (G. antí)	Anti-	Denoting opposite direction.	Antibody
Away from (G. apó)	Apo-	Separated from, derived from, lacking of.	Apophysis
Two-sided (G. amphí)	Amphi-	On both sides, surrounding, double.	Amphipathic
Separation (G. schizó)	Schiz- Schizo-	Denoting split, cleft, division.	Schizophrenia
Rupture (L. hernia)	Hernio-	Combining form relating to hernia.	Herniotomy

Around (G. perí)	Peri-	Denoting around, about.	Pericolitis
Around (L. circum)	Circum- Circun-	Denoting a circular movement, or a position surrounding the part indicated by the word to which it is joined.	Circumanal
Outside of (G. éxo)	Exo-	Meaning exterior, external, outward.	Exocytosis
Outside of (G. éktos)	Ect- Ecto-	Denoting outer, on the outside	Ectoparasite
Outside of (L. extra)	Extra-	Meaning without, outside of.	Extracellular fluid
Within (G. éndon)	End- Endo- Ent- Ento-	Indicating within, inner, absorbing, containing.	Endophyte
Within (L. intra)	Intra-	Meaning within.	Intradermoreaction
Between (L. inter)	Inter-	Meaning between or among.	Interparietal fissure
Left (L. laevus)	Levo-	Denoting left, towards or on the left side.	Levorotatory
Right (L. dexter)	Dextr- Dextro-	Prefixes meaning right, or toward or on the right side.	Dextroduction
Middle (G. mésos)	Mes- Meso-	Prefix meaning middle, or mean.	Mesocardium

Over, after (G. meta)	Meta-	Denoting after, subsequent to, behind, or hindmost, or change of form.	Metastasis
Beginning, origin (G. árcho)	Arch- Archi-	Denoting the first, primitive, ancestral.	Archicerebelum
New (G. neos)	Neo-	Prefix meaning new or recent.	Neocortex
Old (G. palaiós)	Pale- Paleo-	Prefixes meaning old, primitive, primary, early.	Paleocortex
Night (G. nyx nyctós)	Nyct- Nycto-	Combining forms denoting night, nocturnal.	Nyctohemeral rhythm

Quality	*Root, prefix, suffix*	*Meaning*	*Examples of terms*
Same (G. ísos)	Iso-	Meaning equal.	Isogenic
Correct, straight (G. orthós)	Ortho-	Denoting straight, normal or in proper order.	Orthodontist
Smooth (G. leios)	Leio-	Combining form meaning smooth.	Leiodermia
Delicate (G. leptós)	Lept- Lepto-	Combining form meaning light, slender, thin, or frail.	Leptocephaly
Thick (G. pachys)	Pachy-	Prefix denoting thick.	Pachyderma

Slow (G. bradys)	Brady-	Combining form meaning slow.	Bradykinesia
Quick (G. tachys)	Tachy-	Denoting rapid.	Tachycardia
Bent, crooked (G. ankylos)	Ankylo-	Denoting bent, crooked.	Ankylodactyly
Thorny (G. ákantha)	Acantho-	Denoting relationship to a spinous process.	Acanthocyte
Masculine (G. anér andrós)	Andro-	Denoting masculine; pertaining to the male of the species.	Androgenetic alopecia
Solid (G. stereós)	Stereo-	Denoting a solid, or a solid condition or state.	Stereognosis
Hard (G. sklerós)	Scler- Sclero-	Denoting hardness.	Atherosclerosis
Dwarf (G. nános)	Nano-	Combining form relating to dwarfism.	Nanotechnology
Dry (G. xerós)	Xero-	Combining form meaning dry.	Xerophthalmia
Cold (G. psychrós)	Psychro-	Combining form relating to cold.	Psychroalgia
Sweet (G. glykys)	Gluco-	Denoting relationship to glucose.	Glucocerebroside

Quantity	*Root, prefix, suffix*	*Meaning*	*Examples of terms*
More (G. pleíôn)	Pleo-	Denoting more.	Pleocytosis
Excess (G. hypér)	Hyper-	Denoting excessive or above the normal.	Hypercholesteremia
Excess (L. super)	Super-	Denoting excessive or above the normal.	Superacidity
Deficiency (G. hypó)	Hypo-	Denoting deficiency or below the normal.	Hypocalcemia
Deficiency (G. penía)	-penia	Combining form meaning deficiency, poverty.	Neutropenia
Large (G. makrós)	Macro-	Combining form meaning large, long.	Macroblast
Large (G. mégas)	Mega-	Combining form meaning large.	Megacystis
Small (G. mikrós)	Micr- Micro-	Prefixes denoting smallness or microscopic.	Microembolism
Less (G. meión)	Myo-	Combining form meaning less.	Myopia

Light and colour	Root, prefix, suffix	Meaning	Examples of terms
Light (G. phôs)	Phos-	Denoting light.	Phosphorolysis
Colour (G. chróma)	Chrom- Chromat- Chromato- Chromo-	Combining forms meaning colour.	Chromatogram
Grey (G. phaiós)	Pheo-	Combining form meaning dusky, grey, or dun.	Pheochromoblast
Grey (G. poliós)	Polio-	Denoting grey or the grey matter (substantia grisea).	Polioencephalitis
Greyish green (G. glaukós)	Glauc-	Denoting a colour between green and blue.	Glaucoma
Green (G. chlorós)	Chlor- Chloro-	Denoting green; association with chlorine.	Chlorophyll
White (G. leukós)	Leuk- Leuko-	Denoting white.	Leukocyte
White (L. albus)	Alb- Albi-	Denoting white.	Albinism
Black (G. mélas mélanos)	Melan- Melano-	Combining forms meaning black.	Melanemia
Rose (G. rhódon)	Rhod- Rhodo-	Combining forms denoting rose or red colour.	Rhodopsin
Yellow (G. xanthós)	Xanth- Xantho-	Combining forms denoting yellow, yellowish.	Xanthodont

Rainbow (G. îris iridos)	Irid- Irido-	Relating to the iris.	Iridoplegia
Orange (G. kirrós)	Cirr-	Denoting orange colour or relationship to cirrhosis.	Cirrhosis

Shape	*Root, prefix, suffix*	*Meaning*	*Examples of terms*
Shape, form (G. morphé)	Morph- Morpho-	Combining forms relating to shape, form, or structure.	Morphology
Resemblance of form (G. eîdos)	-odes -oid	Suffixes denoting having the form of, like, resembling.	Phyllodes
Stick (G. baktérion)	Bacter-	Denoting bacteria.	Bactericide
Almond (G. Amygdále)	Amygdal-	Denoting the amygdale.	Amygdalectomy
Sphere (G. sphaira)	Sphero-	Denoting spherical; a sphere.	Spherocytosis
Tube (G. sálpigx sálpiggos, meaning tube, trumpet.	Salping- Salpingo-	Combining forms denoting a tube.	Salpingo- ovariotomy
Pipe or tube (G. syrinx)	Syring- Syringo-	Combining forms relating to a syrinx.	Syringospora
Bunch of grapes (G. staphylé)	Staphyl- Staphylo-	Denoting resemblance to a grape or a bunch or grapes.	Staphylococcus

Lentil (G. phakós)	Phaco-	Indicating lens, or relating to a lens.	Phacolysis
Thread (G. nêma nématos)	Nema- Nemat- Nemato-	Combining forms meaning thread, threadlike.	Nematodiasis

Action	*Root, prefix, suffix*	*Meaning*	*Examples of terms*
Stretching (G. ektasis)	-ectasia -ectasis	Combining forms in suffix position used to denote dilatation or expansion.	Lymphangiectasia
Cutting (G. tomos)	-tome -tomy	Combining forms denoting a cutting operation, a cutting instrument.	Crycotomy
Removing (G. ektomé)	-ectomy	Combining form used in suffix position used to denote removal of any anatomical structure.	Vasectomy
Eating (G. phagein)	Phago- -phage -phagia -phagy	Combining forms meaning eating or devouring.	Aerophagy Phagocityze
Loving (G. phileó)	Phylo- -phil -phile -philia -philic	Combining forms denoting affinity for or craving for.	Zoophilia

Fleeing (L. fugo)	-fugal	Suffix denoting movement away from the part indicated by the root of the word.	Corticofugal
Giving birth (G. genés)	-genic	Combining form denoting producing or forming, produced or formed by.	Glucogenic
Making (G. poiésis)	-poiesis	Denoting production.	Hemopoiesis
Sleeping (G. hypnos)	Hypn- Hypno-	Combining forms relating to sleeping or hypnosis.	Hypnology
Benumbing (G. narkoun)	Narco-	Combining form relating to stupor or narcosis.	Narcotic
Moving (G. kinesis)	Kinesi- Kinesio- Kineso- -kinesia	Combining forms relating to motion.	Kinesitherapy Bradykinesia
Speaking (G. lexai)	-lexia -lexis	Combining forms relating to speech.	Dyslexia
Loosening, diluting (G. lysis)	Lys- Lyso- -lysis	Combined forms denoting dissolution.	Lysogenesis Dialysis
Breathing (G. pneó)	Pneo- -pnea	Combining forms denoting breath.	Pneodynamics Tachypnea
Injuring (L. noceo)	Noci-	Combining form relating to hurt, pain, or injury.	Nociceptor

Swelling (G. kélé)	-cele	Denoting a swelling or hernia.	Gastrocele
Smelling (G. osphresis)	Osphresio-	Denoting odour or the sense of semell.	Osphresiology
Seeking (L. peto)	-petal	Suffix denoting movement toward the part indicated by the root of the word.	Centripetal
Falling (G. ptósis)	-ptosis	Suffix denoting a falling or downward displacement of an organ.	Blepharoptosis
Bursting forth (G. rhégnymi)	-rhagia	Suffix denoting excessive or unusual discharge.	Hemorrhagia
Viewing (G. skopeó)	-scopy -scope	Suffix denoting an action or activity involving the use of an instrument for viewing.	Microscope
Stopping (G. states)	-stat	Suffix indicating an agent or instrument intended to keep something from changing or moving.	Thermostat

References

Adab, Beverly (2001) 'The Translation of Advertising: a Framework for Evaluation', *Babel* 47(2): 133-157.

Arnold, Jane (ed.) (1999) *Affect in Language Learning*, Cambridge: Cambridge University Press.

Austin, J.L. (1962) *How To Do Things With Words*, Oxford: Oxford University Press.

Baer, B. J. and G. S. Koby (eds.) (2003) *Beyond the Ivory Tower. Rethinking Translation Pedagogy*, Amsterdam and Philadelphia: John Benjamins. [ATA Scholarly Monograph Series].

Baker, Mona (1992) *In Other Words*, London and New York: Routledge.

Baker, Mona (ed.) (1998) *Encyclopedia of Translation Studies*, London and New York: Routledge.

Balliu, Christian (2001) 'Les traducteurs: ces médecines légistes du texte', *Meta* 46(1): 92-102.

Bastin, Georges (2000 'Evaluating beginners' re-expression and creativity: a positive approach', *The Translator* 6(2): 231-245.

Bazerman, Charles (1998) 'Emerging perspectives on the many dimensions of scientific discourse', in J.R. Martin and Robert Veel (eds) *Reading Science. Critical and Functional Perspectives of Discourses of Science*, London and New York: Routledge, 15-30.

Beylard-Ozeroff, Ann, Jana Králová and Barbara Moser-Mercer (eds) (1998) *Translators' Strategies and Creativity*, Amsterdam and Philadelphia: John Benjamins.

Bhatia, Vijay K. (1993) *Analysing Genre: Language Use in Professional Settings*, London: Longman.

Bowen, Margareta (2000) 'Community Interpreting', *AIIC*, September: 234. [Also available at: http://www.aiic.net/ViewPage.cfm/page234.htm]

Brown, Gillian (1994) 'Modes of understanding', in Gillian Brown, Kirsten Malmkjær, Alastair Pollitt and John Williams (eds) *Language and Understanding,* Cambridge: Cambridge University Press, 9-20.

Gillian Brown, Kirsten Malmkjær, Alastair Pollitt and John Williams (eds) (1994) *Language and Understanding*, Cambridge: Cambridge University Press.

Brown, Theodore L. (2003) *Making truth: Metaphor in Science*, Urbana and Chicago: University of Illinois Press.

Campbell, Stuart (1991) 'Towards a Model of Translation Competence', *Meta* 36(2/3): 329-343.

Candlin, Christopher N. and Ken Hyland (eds) (1999) *Writing: Texts, Processes and Practices*, London and New York: Longman.

Caro, I. and W.B. Stiles (1997) 'Vamos a Traducir los MRV (let's translate the VRM): linguistic and cultural inferences drawn from translating a verbal coding system from English into Spanish', *Psychiatry* 60(3): 233-47.

Cole, P. and J. Morgan (eds) (1975) *Syntax and semantics: Speech acts*, Volume 3, New York: Academia.

Corpas Pastor, Gloria, Adela Martínez García and Mª Carmen Amaya Galván (coords) (2002) *En torno a la traducción-adaptación del mensaje publicitario*, Málaga: Universidad de Málaga.

de Pedro, Raquel (1996) 'Beyond the Words: the Translation of Television Adverts', *Babel* 42(1): 27-45.

Fink, Diana Darley (2002) *Técnicas de lectura rápida*, Bilbao: Deusto.

Fischbach, Henry (1998) *Translation and Medicine*, Amsterdam and Philadelphia: John Benjamins. [ATA Scholarly Monograph Series].

García, Isabel and Vicent Montalt (2002) 'Translating into Textual Genres', *Linguistica Antverpiensia* (Special Issue: *Linguistics and Translation Studies; Translation Studies and Linguistics*), Volume 1, Antwerp: Hoger Institute vor Vertalerse & Tolken, 135-143.

Gardner, Robert, and Wallace E. Lambert (1972) *Attitudes and Motivation in Second Language Acquisition,* Oxford: Oxford University Press.

González Davies, Maria (1998) 'Student Assessment by Medical Specialists, an Experiment in Relating the Undergraduate to the Professional World in the Teaching of Medical Translation in Spain', in Henry Fischbach (ed.) *Translation and Medicine*, Amsterdam and Philadelphia: John Benjamins, 93-102.

------ (2004) *Multiple Voices in the Translation Classroom. Activities, Tasks and Projects*, Amsterdam and Philadelphia: John Benjamins.

González Davies, Maria and Christopher Scott-Tennent (2005) 'A Problem-Solving and Student-Centred Approach to the Translation of Cultural References', *Meta* 50(1): 160-179. [Special issue : *Enseignement de la traduction dans le monde*]

González Davies, Maria, Christopher Scott-Tennent and Fernanda Rodríguez (2001) 'Training in the Application of Translation Strategies for Undergraduate Scientific Translation Students', *Meta* 46(4): 737-744.

Greenhalgh, Trisha (2001) *How to read a paper. The basics of evidence-based medicine,* London: British Medical Journal Books.

Grice, H.P. (1975) 'Logic and Conversation', in P. Cole and J. Morgan (eds) *Syntax and semantics: Speech acts*, Volume 3, New York: Academia, 41-58.

Gutiérrez Roda, B. (1998) *La ciencia empieza en la palabra. Análisis e historia del lenguaje científico,* Barcelona: Península.

Gylys, Barbara A. and Mary Ellen Wedding (2005) *Medical Terminology Systems. A Body Systems Approach*, 5th edition, Philadelphia: F.A. Davies Company.

Hall, Edward T. (1983) *The Dance of Life*, New York: Doubleday.

Hall, G.M. (ed.) *How to Write a Paper*, London: British Medical Journal Books.

Halliday, M.A.K. (1998) 'Things and relations: Rematicising experience as technical knowledge', in J.R. Martin and R. Veel (eds) *Reading Science. Critical and Functional Perspectives of Discourses of Science*, London and New York: Routledge, 185-235.

Hanvey, R.G. (1992) 'Culture', in R.C. Scarcella and R.L. Oxford (eds) *The Tapestry of Language Learning. The Individual in the Classroom,* Boston Mass.: Heinle and Heinle, 182-192.

Hatim, Basil (1997) *Communicating across Cultures*, Exeter: Exeter University Press.

Hatim, Basil and Ian Mason (1990) *Discourse and the Translator*, London: Routledge.

------ (1997) *The Translator as Communicator*, London: Routledge.

Hedge, Tricia (2005) *Writing*, Oxford: Oxford University Press.

Herrell, Adrienne and Michael Jordan (2002) *Active Learning Strategies for Improving Reading Comprehension*, New Jersey and Ohio: Merrill Prentice Hall.

Hervey, Sandor, Ian Higgins and Louise Haywood (1995) *Thinking Spanish Translation*, London and New York: Routledge. [Also, French, Italian, German Translation in the same series]

Huth, Edward J. (1994) *Scientific Style and Format. The CBE Manual for Authors, Editors, and Publishers*, 6th edition, Chicago: CBE.

------ (1999) *Writing and Publishing in Medicine*, Baltimore: Williams and Wilkins.

Jackendoff, R. (1983) *Semantics and Cognition*, Cambridge and London: Massachusetts Institute of Technology.

Jammal, Amal (1999) 'Une méthodologie de la traduction médicale', *Meta* 44(2): 217-237.

Katan, David (1999/2004) *Translating Cultures. An Introduction for Translators, Interpreters and Mediators*, second edition, Manchester: St. Jerome.

Kintsch, Walter (1998) *Comprehension. A Paradigm for Cognition*, Cambridge: Cambridge University Press.

Kiraly, Don (2000) *A Social Constructivist Approach to Translator Education. Empowering the Translator*, Manchester: St. Jerome.

Konstant, Tina (2000) *Speed Reading*, London: Hodder Headline.

Kussmaul, Paul (1995) *Training the Translator*, Amsterdam and Philadelphia: John Benjamins.

Lakoff, George and Mark Johnson (1980) *Metaphors We Live By*, Chicago: University of Chicago Press.

------ (1999) *Philosophy in the Flesh: The Embodied Mind and its Challenge to Western Thought*, New York: Basic Books.

Lee-Jahnke, Hannelore (2001) 'L'enseignement de la traduction médicale au niveau universitaire', *Meta* 46(1): 145-153.

Lent, L., E. Hahn, S. Eremenco, K. Webster and D. Cella (1999) 'Using cross-cultural input to adapt the Functional Assessment of Chronic Illness Therapy (FACIT) scales', *Acta Oncologica*, 695-702.

Márquez, Cristina (2000) 'Entrevista a Fernando Navarro', *Infórmate, Journal of the Spanish of the ATA*, http://www.ata-spd.org/Informate/Entrevistas/fernando_navarro.htm.

Martin, J.R. and R. Veel (eds) (1998) *Reading Science. Critical and Functional Perspectives of Discourses of Science*, London and New York: Routledge.

Massardier-Kenney, Françoise (1998) 'Series Editor's Foreword', in Henry Fischbach (ed.) *Translation and Medicine*, Amsterdam and Philadelphia: John Benjamins.

Matthews, J.R.; J.M. Bowen and R.W. Matthews (2000) *Successful Scientific Writing. A Step-by-Step Guide for the Biological and Medical Sciences,*

Cambridge: Cambridge University Press.

Montalt, Vicent (2005) *Manual de traducció cientificotècnica*, in Biblioteca de Traducció i Interpretació, Vic: Eumo.

Mossop, Brian (2001) *Revising and Editing for Translators*, Manchester: St. Jerome.

Navarro, F. (2005) *Diccionario crítico de dudas inglés-español de dudas de medicina*, Madrid: McGraw-Hill.

Nord, Christiane (1988) *Textanalyse und Übersetzung*, Heidelberg: Groos. English translation by Penelope Sparrow and Christiane Nord (1991) *Text Analysis in Translation*, Amsterdam: Rodopi.

------ (1997) *Translating as a Purposeful Activity*, Manchester: St. Jerome.

Nunan, David (1988) *Syllabus Design*, Oxford: Oxford University Press.

------ (1989) *Designing Tasks for the Communicative Classroom*, Cambridge: Cambridge University Press.

O'Neill, Marla (1998) 'Who Makes a Better Medical Translator: The Medically Knowledgeable Linguist or the Linguistically Knowledgeable Medical Professional? A Physician's Perspective', in Henry Fishbach (ed.) *Translation and Medicine*, Amsterdam and Philadelphia: John Benjamins, 69-80.

Paradis, J.G. and M.L. Zimmerman (1997) *The MIT Guide to Science and Engineering communication*, Cambridge and London: The MIT Press.

Perkes, Courtney (2003) 'A medical speciality in treating Hispanics – New curriculum at UCI will instruct doctors in culture and language', *The Orange County Register*: June 11. [Available at: http://www2.ocregister.com/ocrweb/ocr/article.do?id=43085]

Pilegaard, Morten (1997) 'Translation of medical research articles', in Anna Trosborg (ed.) *Text Typology and Translation*, Amsterdam and Philadephia: John Benjmains, 159-184.

Piotrowska, Maria (1998) 'Towards a Model of Strategies and Techniques for Teaching Translation', in Ann Beylard-Ozeroff, Jana Králová and Barbara Moser-Mercer (eds) *Translators' Strategies and Creativity*, Amsterdam and Philadelphia: John Benjamins, 207-211.

Régent, O. (1992) 'Pratiques de communication en medicine: contextes anglais et français', *Langages* 105: 66-75.

Reiss, Katharina and Hans Vermeer (1984 / 1991) *Grundlegung einer allgemeinen Translationstheorie*, Tübingen: Niemeyer. [*Linguistische Arbeiten* 147]

Sanjuás C., J. Alonso, J. Sanchís, P. Casan, J.M. Broquetas P.J. Ferrie, E.F. Juniper and J.M. Antó (1995) 'Cuestionario de calidad de vida en pacientes con asma: la versión española del Asthma Quality of Life Assessment', *Archivos de Bronconeumología* 31: 219-226.

Scarcella, R.C. and R.L. Oxford (eds) (1992) *The Tapestry of Language Learning. The Individual in the Classroom*, Boston Mass.: Heinle and Heinle.

Scott-Tennent, Christopher and Maria González Davies (forthcoming) 'Effects of Specific Training on the Ability to Deal with Cultural Referents in Translation', *Meta*.

Searle, J.R. (1969) *Speech Acts: An Essay on the Philosophy of Language*, Cambridge: Cambridge University Press.

Segura, Jack (1999) 'The Spanish Language in Medicine', *Translation Journal* 3(3), July. http://accurapid.com/journal/09medic1.htm.

Shackman, Jane (1984) *The Right to be Understood: A Handbook on Working With, Employing and Training Community Interpreters*, Cambridge: National Extension College.

Swales, John M. (1990) *Genre Analysis*, Cambridge: Cambridge University Press.

------ (2000) *English in Today's Research World. A Writing Guide*, Michigan: The University of Michigan Press.

Swales, John M.and C.B. Feak (2004) *Academic Writing for Graduate Students. Essential Tasks and Skills*, Michigan: The University of Michigan Press.

Tatilon, Claude (1990) 'Le texte publicitaire: traduction ou adaptation?', *Meta* 35(1): 243-246.

Trosborg, Anna (ed.) (1997) *Text Typology and Translation*, Amsterdam and Philadephia: John Benjmains.

Victor, David (1992) *International Business Communication*, London: HarperCollins.

Vihla, Minna (1999) *Medical Writing. Modality in Focus*, Amsterdam and Atlanta: Rodopi. [Language and Computers: Studies in practical linguisics]

Wade, Suzanne E. (1990) 'Using think alouds to assess comprehension', *The Reading Teacher* 3: 442-451.

Wakabayashi, Judith (1996) 'Teaching Medical Translation', *Meta* 41(3): 356-365.

Wildsmith, J. (2003) 'How to write a case report', in G.M. Hall (ed.) *How to Write a Paper*, London: British Medical Journal Books, 85-91.

Wilson, Deirdre (1994) 'Relevance and Understanding', in Gillian Brown, Kirsten Malmkjær, Alastair Pollitt and John Williams (eds) *Language and Understanding*, Cambridge: Cambridge University Press, 35-58.

Wright, Patricia (1999) 'Writing and information design of healthcare materials', in Christopher N. Candlin and Ken Hyland (eds) *Writing: Texts, Processes and Practices*, London and New York: Longman, 85-98.

Wright, Sue Ellen and Leland D. Wright, Jr. (eds) (1993) *Scientific and Technological Translation*, Amsterdam and Philadelphia: John Benjamins. [ATA Scholarly Monograph Series].

Index